T0340064

Medical Empiricism and Philosophy of Human Nature in the 17th and 18th Century

Medical Empiricism and Philosophy of Human Nature in the 17th and 18th Century

Edited by

Claire Crignon, Carsten Zelle,
and Nunzio Allocca

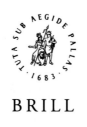

BRILL

LEIDEN | BOSTON

Originally published as Volume XVIII, Nos. 4-5 (2013) of Brill's journal *Early Science and Medicine*.

Cover illustration: Minerva, the personification of *sapientia*, points to the sources of pre-modern sciences: *ratio*, preserved in books, and *experientia* as resource of human senses. This frontispiece (almost completely reproduced here) opens a "Recueil d'expériences et observations sur le combat qui précède du mélange des corps", which collects French translations of three of the most important scientific works of the 17th century: a chemical treatise of Nehemiah Grew, a physiological monograph of Robert Boyle and five articles of Anthony van Leeuwenhoek concerning blood.
The authors and editor would like to thank the Bibliothèque Universitaire de Santé (12 rue de l'école de Médecine, 75005 Paris) and Stéphanie Charreaux for allowing them to use the frontispiece of the following book: Grew, Boyle, Leuwenhoeck, *Recueil d'expériences et observations sur le combat qui précède du mélange des corps*, Paris, E. Michallet, 1679.

Library of Congress Cataloging-in-Publication Data

Medical empiricism and philosophy of human nature in the 17th and 18th century / edited by Claire Crignon, Carsten Zelle, and Nunzio Allocca.
    pages cm
  "Originally published as volume XVIII, nos. 4-5 (2013) of Brill's Journal early science and medicine" --Title page verso.
  Includes bibliographical references and index.
  ISBN 978-90-04-26812-8 (hardback : acid-free paper) -- ISBN 978-90-04-26813-5 (e-book) 1. Medicine--Philosophy. 2. Philosophical anthropology--History. 3. Human body (Philosophy) 4. Medicine--History--17th century. 5. Medicine--History--18th century. I. Crignon, Claire, editor of compilation. II. Zelle, Carsten, 1953, editor of compilation. III. Allocca, Nunzio, editor of compilation.

R723.M363 2013
610.1--dc23   2014001484

This publication has been typeset in the multilingual "Brill" typeface. With over 5,100 characters covering Latin, IPA, Greek, and Cyrillic, this typeface is especially suitable for use in the humanities. For more information, please see www.brill.com/brill-typeface.

ISBN 978 90 04 26812 8 (hardback)
ISBN 978 90 04 26813 5 (e-book)

Contents

> The page numbers in the above table of contents and in the indices refer to the bracketed page numbers in this volume.

Introduction

Claire Crignon, Carsten Zelle, Nunzio Allocca

It may seem surprising to devote an entire book to the question of empiricism and, more specifically, its relation to medicine and philosophy with a special focus on the seventeenth and eighteenth centuries.

The adjective 'empirical' is used to denote a medical school that flourished over the course of the late Hellenistic period and at the beginning of the Roman Empire along with the 'dogmatic' and 'methodic' schools.[1] The school of the 'empirics' was characterised by a rejection of looking for causes, giving precedence instead to the treatment of illnesses based on the observation of symptoms. Refusing the assistance of reason in aiming to discover hidden causes, practitioners trusted only those things that are obvious to senses. Indeed, as Pierre Pellegrin stresses, their position is often seen as a critical interrogation of the metaphysical pretensions of reason.[2]

At the beginning of the modern period, the term was used in a pejorative way. In Bacon's works, for example, the adjective refers more broadly to a blind practice of science: the science of the 'empiricists'," who behave like ants ("the manner of the ant"), as they content themselves with gathering empirical data without any effort towards rationalism. This practice lies in opposition to philosophy which, according to the

---

[1] Heinrich von Staden, "Hairesis and Heresy: The Case of the *haireseis iatrikai*," in Ben F. Meyer, ed., *Jewish and Christian Self-Definition*, vol. 3. *Self-Definition in the Graeco-Roman World* (London, 1982), 76-100. See also Jackie Pigeaud, "Les écoles médicales à Rome," in Pigeaud, ed., *Actes du 2ᵉ colloque international sur les textes médicaux latins antiques* (Geneva, 1991).

[2] See Pierre Pellegrin, "Le débat des écoles médicales sur la médecine et le savoir médical," in Galien, *Traités philosophiques & logiques*, transl. Pellegrin et al. (Paris, 1998), Introduction, 32-62, esp. 37.

author of the *Novum Organum* (1620), must be founded on an alliance between experience and reason ("the manner of the bee").[3]

The emergence of the term 'empiricism' as a noun denoting a philosophical school of thought occurs much later. We may recall that it was in fact Kant who gave birth to this notion in the *Critique of Pure Reason* in 1781.[4] Kant considers the attitude of the "empiricist philosopher" as fecund insofar as it dismisses "the indiscrete curiosity and presumption of reason" and prohibits that one should "permit himself to seek a cause beyond nature."[5] Kant thus gives Hume credit for demonstrating the need for a complete study of the claims of pure reason but at the same time deplores the fact that his empiricism has led to a "scepticism" which has impinged on "any theoretical use of reason."[6] In contrast to rationalism, empiricism was from that point onwards also associated with scepticism and considered a form of the renunciation of knowledge.

This characterisation of empiricism by Kant has played an important role in the creation of a certain number of fixed ideas or 'myths' about empiricism.[7] As Guido Giglioni notes about Bacon ("Learning to Read Nature: Francis Bacon's Notion of Experiential Literacy"), empiricism was often mistaken for an epistemological position and at the same time as an ontological affirmation. The position that the whole of our knowledge has a sensible starting point, however, does not necessarily lead us to claim that reality is in itself unknowable. Widely divergent philosophies have thus been grouped under the same heading. Indeed, what is the common link between Bacon's position in the *Novum Organum*— that it is possible to acquire knowledge of "latent schematism in bodies," of the "forms" of natural things[8]—and Locke's position when he shares,

---

3) Francis Bacon, *Novum Organum* I, 95, in *The Oxford Francis Bacon*, Graham Rees and Maria Wakely eds., vol. XI (Oxford, 2004), 153.

4) Cf. [Art.] "Empirismus," in Joachim Ritter et al., eds., *Historisches Wörterbuch der Philosophie*, vol. 2 (Darmstadt, 1972), 477–78.

5) Immanuel Kant, *Kritik der reinen Vernunft*, Transcendental Dialectic, Bk. II, chap. II, 3 (= Akademieausgabe, vol. 3, 326-27).

6) Immanuel Kant, *Kritik der praktischen Vernunft*, Ist part, bk. II, ch. I, 2 (= Akademieausgabe, vol. 5, 52).

7) David Fate Norton, "The Myth of British Empiricism," *History of European Ideas*, vol. I (1981), 331-44.

8) Francis Bacon, *Novum Organum*, bk. II, aph. 7, in Graham Rees & Maria Wakely, eds., *The Oxford Francis Bacon*, vol. XI (Oxford, 2004), 211.

in his medical texts, his doubts about the possibility of acquiring a knowledge of the operations through which nature accomplishes its operations in the body via anatomy? As Locke writes, "Now it is certain and beyond controversy that nature perform all her operations in the body by parts so minute and insensible that I think no body will ever hope or pretend, even by the assistance of glasses or any other invention to come to a sight of them (...)."[9]

Kant cannot of course be considered the sole person responsible for the excessively uniform view we have of empiricism or for the sometimes over-simplistic opposition between a 'rationalist' philosophical school of thought (of which Descartes or Leibniz would be eminent representatives) and an 'empirical' philosophical school of thought (from Bacon to Hume).[10] This opposition influences how we read the texts from the modern period in question, a reading that the contributions gathered here invite us to challenge. In particular, the tendency to read metaphysical texts relating to the status of body, to the living or to the relations between spirit and body separate from the medical treatises, manuscripts and letters exchanged between philosophers and physicians in the seventeenth and eighteenth centuries is called into question. This is what, in our eyes, has justified the need to return to the close relations established between medicine and natural philosophy at the beginning of the modern period in order to question anew the relations between reason and experience and to demonstrate to a broader degree how the debates between the authors, presented as 'rationalists' or 'empiricists', are essential for recounting the birth of the concept of empiricism itself.

***

The contributions gathered in this volume endeavour to evaluate the role played by medical empiricism in the emergence of a philosophy of human nature in the seventeenth century and the role played by philosophical anthropology in the eighteenth century. They question the position of medicine within so-called "natural philosophy," which encompasses physiology and anatomy, as well as physics, astronomy and chemistry.

---

9) John Locke, *Anatomia*, PRO, 30/24/47/2, f. 31r.
10) See Hans Jürgen Engfer, *Empirismus versus Rationalismus. Kritik eines philosophischen Schemas* (Paderborn, 1996).

There is tension, however, specifically between the goals pursued by the "natural philosopher" and the objectives set by the physician. Within natural philosophy, the primary goal is to know nature, the body and the living, and this knowledge implies an effort to understand the causes of natural phenomena. For the physician, on the other hand, the primary goal is to cure the patients' bodies as they are presented to him. These activities are initially guided by a pragmatic objective. The empiricist physician, as described by Galen, does not categorically reject the aim of discovering the causes of illnesses, but instead gives priority to curing the sick, subordinating the theoretical search for causes to this practical goal. If empiricist physicians do not advocate dissection, it is because they consider that it is not "necessary to the medical art."[11] The physicians' competences should not be judged by theoretical reasoning but instead by their ability to restore their patients to health:

> Why, then, should anyone believe rather in Hippocrates than in Herophilus, why in him rather than in Asclepiades? If one wants to be guided by reasoning, they go on, the reasoning of all of them can appear not improbable; if by method of treatment, all of them have restored sick folk to health: therefore one ought not to derogate from anyone's credit, either in argument or in authority. Even philosophers would have become the greatest of medical practitioners, if reasoning from theory could have made them so.[12]

This tension between natural philosophy and medicine is present throughout the modern period (see our first section: "The Dispute between Metaphysics and Empiricism"). How should we evaluate the interest accorded by some philosophers to medical observations and experiments? Should we place metaphysical considerations about the nature of the body and practical observations about particular bodies on opposing sides? As Anne-Lise Rey shows ("The Status of Leibniz's Medical Experiments: A Provisional Empiricism?"), we should rather try to articulate and think about these various aspects together, through one philosophical understanding. This allows us to understand how empiricism may be sometimes thought of as something "provisional" and al-

---

[11] Galen, *On the Sects for Beginners*, in Richard Walzer & Michael Frede, transl., *Three Treatises on the Nature of Science* (Indianapolis, 1985), ch. 5.
[12] Celsus, *De Medicina*, transl. Walter George Spencer (London, 1935), Preamble.

lowing for the discovery of a "foretaste of knowledge to come." But the tension may be stronger. Empiricism can be used within opposing metaphysical strategies: to demonstrate empirically the action of the spirit (cf. the article by Claire Etchegaray on Whytt) or to show the necessity of materialism. Besides, as Claire Crignon highlights, some "Modern philosophical readings of classical medical empiricism" renew the critical interrogation of a metaphysical use of reason. Medicine plays here a very important role in the distinction established between natural philosophy in its *speculative* manifestation (the aim of reason is to know things, to discover the causes of phenomena) and in its *experimental* manifestation (the aim of medicine is to cure patients, even if we ignore the causes of the disease).[13]

The argument of therapeutic efficacy, however, is a double-edged sword. Those who promise patients miraculous recoveries and dispense with any attempt to gain knowledge of nature are, in fact, considered to be charlatans and impostors. In his *Advancement of Learning* of 1605, Bacon already condemned the "weakness and credulity of men" that led them to "preferre a montabanke or Witch, before a learned Physitian."[14] In his *Cyclopedia*, published in 1728, Ephraim Chambers notes that "(...) the word empiric is now more odious than ever, being confounded with that of a charlatan or quack, and applied to persons who practise physic at random, or understanding any thing of the principles of the art."[15] Before the emergence of the term as a noun, the adjective 'empiric' was used to qualify a non-methodical and non-scientific form of medical practice. In Friedrich Hoffmann's view, for example, unreflective empiricism has pejorative connotations. According to him, a "reasonable physician" should have the ability to observe and to analyse; i.e. "not to proceed *empirice*, but *methodice*."[16]

---

[13] Peter Anstey, "Experimental versus Speculative Natural Philosophy," in Peter Anstey & John A. Schuster, eds., *The Science of Nature in Seventeenth Century. Patterns of Change in Early Natural Philosophy* (Dordrecht, 2005), 215-42.

[14] Francis Bacon, *The Advancement of Learning*, in Michael Kiernan, ed., *The Oxford Francis Bacon*, vol. IV, 97 (Oxford, 2000).

[15] Ephraim Chambers, *Cyclopedia, or, An universal dictionary of arts and sciences*, vol. II (London, 1728), 303.

[16] Friedrich Hoffmann, *Medicina Consultatoria: Worinnen unterschiedliche über einige schwehre Casus ausgearbeitete Consilia, auch Responsa Facultatis Medicæ enthalten [...]*, 12 vols. (Halle, 1721-1739), vol. 9, 1732, Preface, fol. 3r.

It is precisely to distinguish themselves from this pejorative meaning of empiricism that modern physicians returned to the ancient meaning of medical empiricism as it had been defined since Celsus and Galen. James Primerose recalls in his *De vulgi in medicina erroribus* (1638) that the "Empyricks in times past were very learned and skilfull men," who were not content to offer remedies haphazardly and in keeping with past successes, but instead based their practice on rules and a method: "they followed a certain method, or rather an order in curing (...)."[17]

This explains why authors such as Bacon, Boyle, Sydenham and Hoffmann explicitly refer to the Hippocratic method of observation to demonstrate how it is possible to infer a certain number of principles or theorems based on the "visible" or "obvious" causes offered by experience. Contrary to this, the Galen tradition was judged in a very harsh light. Hoffmann wrote in his case collection:

> Der *Hippocrates* hat gewiß hierinnen sehr klüglich gehandelt und ist sonderlich zu rühmen, daß er sich mehr um *observationes* bekümmert, als sich auf *raisonnements* geleget. *Galenus* hingegen war ein *raisonneur*, und sahe sich wenig nach *observationibus* um, sondern bemühete sich vielmehr die Wirckungen der Natur in seine *speculationes* einzuschliessen, und aus seinem eigenen Kopffe eine *theorie* zu schmieden.[18]

The observation and classification of illnesses, then, takes precedence over the search for causes (see section III: "Relevance of Case Studies"). As Gianna Pomata and Nancy Siraisi have shown, case histories and autopsy narratives belong to *historia*, a genre which is not only characteristic of civil history but also used to refer to practices of descriptions and observation in natural history and medicine: "When Fabricius of Acquapadente or William Harvey, for instance, wrote the results of their anatomical investigations, they regularly started with what they called a *historia*, meaning a thorough description of the structure of bodily parts preliminary to the understanding of their function or use."[19] As Peter

---

[17] James Primerose, Robert Wittie, transl., *Populars Errours. Or the Errours of the People in Physick* (London, 1651), ch. VI, "Of Mountibanks," 22-23.

[18] Hoffmann, *Medicina Consultatoria*, vol. 3, 1723, Preface „Von dem Nutzen guter *Observationum* und Schaden der falschen *Theorie in praxi medica*," fol. 4v.

[19] See *Historia, Empiricism and Erudition in Early Modern Europe*, Gianna Pomata & Nancy G. Siraisi, eds. (Cambridge, MA, 2005), Introduction, 2-3.

Dear points out, "a generally Baconian sense of natural history remained particularly important in English natural philosophy, including that of the early Royal Society, for the rest of the century."[20] But this trend is limited neither to England nor to the seventeenth century. We may, for example, follow during the eighteenth century, in Germany, the emergence of new forms of observation that were turned towards the physicians themselves (the "self-observation" of the "reasonable physicians" suggested by Carsten Zelle in section III). Observation also played a crucial role in the birth of a very specific genre of medical writing, medical periodicals, which consisted of collections of cases and observations (cf. Yvonne Wübben, "Writing Case Studies" in section III).

Modern medical empiricism, however, adopts a very different face, both practical and methodical, and the reference to ancient empiricism often works in a critical way. On the one hand, anatomists reproach the observation practiced by Hippocrates for remaining too passive and not really serving to cure the sick. The argument of therapeutic efficacy begins to be used to advocate a more active form of empiricism, authorizing a shift towards dissection and experimentation as the only ways of investigating the knowledge passed on by the ancients in a critical manner and examining things themselves instead of referring to the ancients' books: "And hence it is, that without the due admonition of the senses, without frequent observation and reiterated experiment, our mind goes astray after phantoms and appearances."[21] On the other hand, the revival of anatomy which began at the end of the Renaissance and the resulting discussions about method moved the debate onto an epistemological level and not just a therapeutic one. In the tradition of Vesalius and then Harvey, the new anatomists proposed a genetic model of knowledge,[22] insisting on the necessity of questioning things themselves, beginning with the perception of individual things offered to the

---

[20] Peter Dear, "The Meanings of Experience," in Katherine Park & Lorraine Daston, eds., *The Cambridge History of Science,* vol. 3: *Early Modern Science* (Cambridge, 2006), 116.

[21] William Harvey, *Anatomical Exercises on the Generation of Animals,* in R, Maynard Hutchins, ed., *Great Books of the Western World, Gilbert, Galileo, Harvey* (Chicago, 1952), Introduction, 333.

[22] André Charrak, *Empirisme et Théorie de la Connaissance. Réflexion et fondement des sciences au XVIIIᵉ siècle* (Paris, 2009).

senses ("embracing nature with our own eyes"[23]), in order to progress towards knowledge of universal matters. At the same time, the tension between the diversity of natural phenomena observed by means of comparative anatomy and the uniformity of nature's rules makes it difficult to generalise knowledge, as shown in Domenico Bertoloni Meli's article on the anatomy of plants and insects by Malpighi ("Of Snails and Horsetails" in section II).

Ultimately, it is the specificity of modern empiricism compared with ancient empiricism that is at the heart of the reciprocal exchanges between anatomical research, observation and classification on the one hand, and philosophical reflection on the knowledge of causes, on the diversity and unity of nature and the passing from the particular to the universal on the other. In fact, it is in no way certain that a common denominator between all the authors and all the doctrines that identify with the empiricism of the seventeenth and eighteenth centuries can be found. As Bas Van Fraassen notes, empiricism is characterised not by defending "theses" but instead by adopting attitudes or "stances."[24] We do not have here a theoretical position or body of knowledge, but instead different kinds of "arts of empirical research" (Section II) or different kinds of "empirical gestures." Empiricism has many different faces: it may be decried as a non-scientific practice or advocated as a method requiring an alliance with reason; it may claim to be affiliated with Hippocrates' observation method and take the form of a phenomenalistic rendering of empiricism, or recommend that things themselves be put to the test by turning to experience as "peira," a trial or test, a critical instance of sharing and decision. As Philippe Hamou suggested in his summary of the debates proposed at the end of the trilateral workshop which assembled a joint German, Italian and French team at Villa Vigoni in May 2011, it is less about an "essence" of medical and philosophical empiricism and more a series of specifically modern "acts."

The first such act involves abandoning books in order to dedicate oneself to dissecting nature, advocated by Harvey in the *epistle dedicatory* on

---

[23] "(...) the comprehension of universals by understanding is based upon the perception of individual things by the senses." Harvey, *Anatomical Exercises*, 332; Harvey, *An Anatomical Disputation concerning the Movement of the Heart and Blood in Living Creatures* (1628), transl. Gweneth Whitteridge (Oxford, 1976), 29
[24] Bas C. Van Fraassen, *The Empirical Stance* (New Haven, 2002).

the treatise on blood circulation: "(...) I do not profess either to learn or teach anatomy from books or from the maxims of philosophers, but from dissections and from the fabric of Nature herself."[25] This is an act that assumes recognition of the diversity of phenomena observed and invites us to make comparisons (comparative anatomy). It is an act that also implies the recognition of nature as more subtle than our senses and, thus, of the need to turn to instruments: the microscope of nature (Domenico Bertoloni Meli), the real microscope or a virtual microscope.

The second is the affirmation of the superior and independent authority of the senses which implies an acceptance of what they show us, even if it is contrary to what understanding suggests and leads to an act of breaking away from the ancients.

The third act means turning attention towards the particular and the individual (the diversity of species and individuals, the particularity of cases) which, in this case, for the physician, concerns treating a *sick person* rather than an illness and reinforces the legitimacy of these acts. As Thomas Willis explains in his preface to *Of Fevers* (1659), it is in "sitting oftentimes by the Sick," in endeavouring to "weigh all the symptoms, and to put them, with exact Diaries of the Diseases, into Writing" that he "began to adapt general Notions from particular Events." The observation of "accidents and courses of fevers" and the taking into consideration of the mortality rate caused by the illness ("a disease by which the third part of Mortals have still Fallen to this day") forbid physicians "to shut their Eyes and remain blind in the Light it self."[26]

The fourth and final act is the priority given to a clinical description of the patient's nature, the history of the illness, an indication of the treatments used and the outcome of the illness over explanation. This is an act which leads the physician to refer to the art of portraiture, as was demonstrated at our conference with regard to Sydenham, who could brush aside hypotheses in order to concentrate on observing more particular details:

---

[25] William Harvey, *Anatomical Disputation Concerning the Movement of the Heart and Blood in Living Creatures*, Epistle Dedicatory to Dr. Argent, transl. Gweneth Whitteridge (Oxford, 1976) 7, see also ch. 1, 29.

[26] Thomas Willis, The Preface to the *Treatise of Fevers* (1659), in *Dr. Willis's Practice of Physick, Being the Whole Works*, transl. Samuel Pordage (London, 1684), 45.

In writing the history of a disease, every philosophical hypothesis whatsoever, that has previously occupied the mind of the author, should lie in abeyance. This being done, the clear and natural phenomena of the disease should be noted—these, and these only. They should be noted accurately, and in all their minuteness; in imitation of the exquisite industry of those painters who represent in their portraits the smallest moles and the faintest spots.[27]

**

This volume is based on talks given during the first (May 2011, 9-12) of a series of three workshops devoted to "Reshaping Man: Medical Discoveries and Philosophies of Human Nature, German Empire, Italy, France, Great Britain, seventeenth and eighteenth Centuries." The aim of this research project, which brings together German, Italian and French researchers, was to understand the constitution of a modern image of man and to study its transformations, starting from the debate between physicians and philosophers, which was revived in the new human and animal anatomy and physiology according to Vesalius.

Villa Vigoni (Centro Italo-Tedesco per l'Eccellenza Europea / Deutsch-Italienisches Zentrum für Europäische Excellenz in Loveno di Menaggio, Italy) is an institution devoted to the promotion of European research. It offers a unique and beautiful location for research as well as the time and leisure, which are too often missing, to establish ties and develop collaborative research projects between different teams and schools of thought. Carsten Zelle (Ruhr-Universität Bochum), Nunzio Allocca (Roma, Sapienza—Università di Roma), Claire Crignon (Paris IV, Sorbonne), Stefanie Buchenau (Paris VIII, Saint-Denis) and Anne-Lise Rey (Lille I) played an active role in the organisation of the conference. It was supported by the Deutsche Forschungsgemeinschaft, Villa Vigoni, the Fondation Maison des Sciences de l'Homme, the ANR Jeune Chercheur Philomed (Université Paris VIII) and the French Embassy in Italy. We are very grateful for the support received and the material assistance provided by Villa Vigoni.

---

[27] Thomas Sydenham, *Medical Observations Concerning the History and Cure of Acute Diseases*, in Robert Gordon Latham, ed., *The Works of Thomas Sydenham* (London, 1850), vol. 1, Preface to the third edition (1666), § 9.

I. THE DISPUTE BETWEEN METAPHYSICS AND EMPIRICISM

The Debate about *methodus medendi* during the Second Half of the Seventeenth Century in England: Modern Philosophical Readings of Classical Medical Empiricism in Bacon, Nedham, Willis and Boyle

Claire Crignon
*Université Paris IV/ Sorbonne**

Abstract

Following a recent trend in the field of the history of philosophy and medicine, this paper stresses the necessity of recognizing empiricism's patent indebtedness to the sciences of the body. While the tribute paid to the Hippocratic method of observation in the work of Thomas Sydenham is well known, it seems necessary to take into account a trend more critical of ancient medicine developed by followers of chemical medicine who considered the doctrine of elements and humours to be a typical example of the idols that hinder the improvement of medical knowledge and defend the necessity of experimentation (comparative anatomy, dissection, autopsy, chemical analysis of bodies). In light of the fact that modern discoveries (blood circulation, the lymphatic system, theory of fevers) resulted in a "new frame of human nature," they developed a critical reading of ancient empiricism. As a consequence, we can distinguish between two distinct anti-speculative traditions in the genesis of philosophical empiricism. The first (which includes Bacon, Boyle and Willis) recommends an active investigation into nature and refers to the figure of Democritus, the ancient philosopher who devoted himself to the dissection of beasts. Defenders of this first tradition refuse point-blank to be called 'empiricists', a label which had a very negative meaning during the seventeenth century, when it was used to dismiss charlatans and quacks. The other tradition (including Sydenham and Locke), stressing as it does the role of description and observation, is more sceptical of the ability of dissection or anatomy to give us access to causes of diseases. This later tradition comes closer to the definition of ancient empiricism and to the figure of Hippocrates.

* Université Paris Sorbonne, UFR de Philosophie, 1 rue Victor Cousin, 75005 Paris (claire. crignon@paris-sorbonne.fr). I would like to thank Thomas Swan for his reading and corrections of the English version of this text and Philippe Hamou for his critical observations on this paper.

Keywords

ancient empiricism, modern empiricism, quacks, observation, experimental philosophy, speculative philosophy, medicine, humorism, chemical medicine, corpuscularism, blood circulation, fevers, human nature, Francis Bacon, William Harvey, Marchamont Nedham, Thomas Willis, Robert Boyle, Thomas Sydenham, Celsus, Galen, Hippocrates, Democritus

1. Introduction

The aversion of English philosophers towards what they called "speculative philosophy" or "a systematic way of writing" are well known, as is the concomitant development of experimental philosophy, which followed Bacon's call to build knowledge without rejecting experience and starting from a true dissection of the world.[1] But do we always know what we are talking about when we use the label of 'empiricism' to define the modern English philosophical tradition from Bacon to Locke? Philosophical labels are useful, but they may also hide conceptual vagueness.

One way to overcome this vagueness is to focus on empirical research in the sciences (physics, astronomy, optics, chemistry, etc.) and to try and understand its role in the emergence of the 'experimental method' promoted and supported by philosophers and scientists taking part in the creation of the Royal Society in 1660.[2] Moreover, we may also underline the crucial importance of one field of research in the genesis of what we call an 'empiricist' conception of knowledge. As François Duchesneau has shown, it would be difficult to understand Locke's conception of the links between experience and reason if one did not start from his medical formation and if we did not keep in mind the method of observation developed by his contemporary and collaborator, the physician Thomas Sydenham.[3] More recently, Charles T. Wolfe and Ofer Gal have under-

---

[1] Bacon, *Novum Organum* I, 124, in Graham Rees and Lisa Jardine, eds., *The Oxford Francis Bacon*, vol. XII (Oxford, 2004). On this distinction between speculative and experimental philosophy, see Peter Anstey, "Experimental versus Speculative Natural Philosophy," in Peter R. Anstey and John A. Schuster, eds., *The Science of Nature in the Seventeenth Century: Patters of Change in Early Modern Natural Philosophy* (Dordrecht, 2005), 215-42.

[2] See Michael Ben–Chaim, *Experimental Philosophy and the Birth of Empirical Science: Boyle, Locke, and Newton* (Ashgate, 2004).

[3] François Duchesneau, *L'empirisme de Locke* (The Hague, 1973), VII.

lined the necessity to "re-embody our understanding of empiricism" and to recognize "empiricism's patent indebtedness to the sciences of the body—medicine, physiology, natural history and chemistry."[4]

The sciences of the body, however, took various forms during the seventeenth century. Humorism and the Galenic conception of the body were still going strong, even if these traditional explanations of the origin of natural things was challenged by the rise of chemical medicine (with the work of Paracelsus and Van Helmont) and, at the same time, by the emergence of mechanism and corpuscularism. Medicine was as a battlefield during this period in which the contenders appealed to various definitions of experience.[5] Followers of chemical medicine and of Van Helmont presented themselves as the champions of observation and experimentation but expressed a strong rejection of Hippocratic empirical method of observation.[6] In addition, the word 'empiric' was used in a highly polemical way in the field of medicine to designate those who "practice physick at random" without any method, "charlatans" or "quacks."[7] As Ephraïm Chambers notes in his *Cyclopedia*, this use of the label serves "those physicians servilely attached to the train and method of the schools, the reasonings of Hippocrates and Galien" against those "who think more freely, and are less devoted to antiquity,"[8] i.e., against chemical physicians but also against all those who defended the necessity of grounding scientific discoveries in experimentation.

The aim of this paper is to show that we must take into consideration this highly polemical context if we want to understand the variety of anti-speculative medical traditions which played an important role in the genesis of modern philosophical empiricism. I will focus here on the

---

4) Charles T. Wolfe and Ofer Gal, eds., *The Body as Object and Instrument of Knowledge, Embodied Empiricism in Early Modern Science* (Dordrecht, 2010), 2.

5) Harold J. Cook, *The Decline of the Old Medical Regime in Stuart London* (Ithaca, NY, and London, 1986).

6) It is important to point out the fact that these various and antagonistic explanations of the natural functions often cohabit one and the same work. See, for example, recent research on the influence of Helmontian medicine upon Locke's conception of medical art: Peter Anstey, "John Locke and Helmontian Medicine," in Wolfe and Gal, eds., *The Body*, 93-117.

7) Ephraïm Chambers, *Cyclopedia, or, An universal dictionary of arts and sciences* (London, 1728), II, 303.

8) *Ibid.*

debate surrounding the definition of a new method in medicine (*metho-dus medendi*) which followed the important discoveries that were made at the beginning of the seventeenth century (especially blood circulation). Underlining the fact that these discoveries revealed a new "human frame"[9] some physicians and natural philosophers expressed doubts about the validity of a method (the Hippocratic one) that was based on an outdated characterization of human nature. One way to discredit this method was to show that it was obnoxious to the practice of medicine, conducive to the neglect of the relief of the patient and that it contributed to the success of "empiricks physicians" (i.e., "quacks"). The necessity of proving that empiricism can constitute a true method and is not incompatible with an investigation into the causes of diseases pushed modern philosophers (Bacon, Willis and Boyle) towards finding alternative models or figures in the ancient history of medicine. Democritus, as we will see, was one of these alternative figures who were used to defend modern discoveries (like Harvey's) and explain, at the same time, the difficulty in accepting it.

2. A New Frame of Human Nature?

It is not without reason that the English physician Thomas Sydenham (1624–1689) was called by his contemporaries "the English Hippocrates." In the preface to his *Observationes Medicae*, published in 1676, Sydenham pays tribute to the Hippocratic method of observation.[10] "History of all diseases," on the one hand, and "a fixed and complet method of cure," on the other, are the best ways to struggle against vain hypotheses and speculative philosophy.[11] Sydenham also reminds us how Francis Bacon re-

---

9) See Thomas Willis, "A Medical-Philosophical Discourse of Fermentation," in *Dr Willis Practice of Physick, Being the Whole Works* (London, 1684).

10) "The Performances of the antients in this science, and chiefly of Hippocrates, are well known (...)." *The Entire Works of Dr. Thomas Sydenham, newly made English from the Originals, wherein the History of acute and chronic Diseases and the safest and most effectual Methods of treating them, are faithfully, clearly, and accurately delivered*, transl. John Swan (London, 1742), The Author's Preface, § 3, II.

11) 'Hypothesis' means here a supposed principle not necessarily connected to experience.

grets, in the second book of his *Advancement of Learning*, the abandonment of the Hippocratic method, calling upon physicians to start from a serious and attentive history of diseases.[12] We do not find, by Sydenham's pen, a strong emphasis upon recent medical discoveries.[13] Moreover, we know that, as with Locke, he expresses some distrust towards anatomical practice and its ability to give us knowledge of physical bodies.[14] The Hippocratic method of observation and description of diseases appears as the best way to avoid empty and speculative hypotheses. While this revival of Hippocratism during the second half of the seventeenth century is well known, we should not forget that earlier, in the middle of the century, there was a very strong opposition to the idea that the Hippocratic method should play a role in the reform and progress of the medical art. The English polemist Marchamond Nedham, for example, published at the end of 1664 a treatise devoted to the "renovation of the art of Physick," entitled *Medela Medicinae. A Plea for the free Profession and a Renovation of the Art of Physick*.[15] Remaining close to chemical medicine and to the doctrine of Van Helmont, Nedham shows himself to be very critical towards classical medical doctrines and strongly rejects humorism.[16] Let us remember that he wrote this pamphlet at the very moment when the Society of Chymical Physitians was trying to establish itself against the influence of the Royal Society of Physicians and against what Harold J. Cook has called "the old medical regime."[17] This polemical context explains the need to present the ancient medical tradition as

---

[12] Francis Bacon, *The Advancement of Learning*, in Graham Rees and Lisa Jardine, eds., *The Oxford Francis Bacon*, vol. IV (Oxford, 2000), 99.

[13] Sydenham, *Medical Observations*, in *The Entire Works of Dr. Th. Sydenham*, The Author's preface, § 3, II (emphasis added).

[14] See Peter Anstey, *John Locke and Natural Philosophy* (Oxford, 2010), esp. ch. 2, 31-45. See also Locke's medical manuscripts, *Anatomia* (1668) and *De Arte Medica* (1669) [PRO 30/24/47/2].

[15] On Nedham, see Cook, *The Decline*, 145. See also Lester S. King, *The Road to Medical Enlightenment, 1650–1695* (New York, 1970), 145-54.

[16] Concerning Van Helmont's rejection of Galenical thought and humorism and the diffusion of his thought in seventeenth-century English natural philosophy, see Antonio Clericuzio, "Les débuts de la carrière de Boyle, l'iatrochimie helmontienne et le cercle de Hartlib," in Myriam Dennehy and Charles Ramond, eds., *La philosophie naturelle de Robert Boyle* (Paris, 2009), 47-70.

[17] See note 5.

conservative and needless. Far from being presented as the father of medical art, according to Nedham, Hippocrates's thought must be considered an "idol," which obstructs men's minds. In fact, this doctrine had already been rejected by the genuine father of medicine, the new Hippocrates, William Harvey, in his *Treatise on the Generation of Animals* (London, 1651): "He [Hippocrates] may be called the Father of the Four Elements, and of the Four Phansies called Humours, which *our Hippocrates* (as some call him) Dr. Harvey approves not (De Gen Animal exercit. 52), and allows but one."[18]

Nedham's intention in this polemical treatise, which attacks the partisans of ancient medicine and hails the defenders of the new chemical doctrines, is to pay tribute to those modern physicians and anatomists, like Thomas Willis and William Digby in England, but also Thomas Bartholin, Sylvius de la Boe and Regius[19] in Holland, who reject "Galenick principles" and "rebuild Physick from the very ground" using "sensible experiments."[20] Using their "own industry" and trusting only their "own eyes and observations," they have brought about a "new frame of human nature"[21] and convinced us that diseases could no longer be explained using the four principles of the Hippocratico-Galenic doctrine. For Nedham, those who defend the "old medical doctrines" propose "a Philosophy and Physick formed up of Intellectual Conceptions, digested into Conclusions and Aphorisms," which will encourage the rise of "Idols and Phantasies" instead of making the senses the best guides to establish a certain truth.[22] According to him, an active observation of nature, which gives priority to the senses, uses comparative anatomy and proceeds to tests and trials (such as chemical decomposition of natural bodies) is the

---

[18] Emphasis added. Nedham, *Medela Medicinae* (London, 1665), 2. Nedham refers to the 52th exercitation of Harvey's *Treatise on Generation*, where Harvey qualifies "the blood as prime element in the body" and explicitly rejects humorism. William Harvey, *On the Generation of Animals*, in *The Works of William Harvey*, ed., Robert Willis (London, 1847), 379-89.

[19] According to Nedham, Regius has "improved the cartesian principles." See his praise of Regius's *Natural Philosophy*: Nedham, *Medela Medicina*, 13.

[20] "(...) sensible experiment the best guide to philosophy and physick," Nedham, *Medela Medicina*, 235-36.

[21] *Ibid.*, 204.

[22] *Ibid.*, 235.

only way to rebuild 'physick' and the therapeutic method upon new foundations.

Nedham gives special attention to modern discoveries and especially to Harvey's discovery of blood circulation. But what is it that allows him to present Harvey as a "new Hippocrates"?[23] To justify this polemical assertion, he uses the work of Thomas Willis, physician and "Professor of Natural Philosophy" at Oxford,[24] one of "the Ornament of our nation next to immortal Harvey" and quotes his preface to the *Treatise of Feavers*, first published in Latin in 1659.[25] This text is indeed crucial to understanding how medical observations and discoveries have been used by modern anatomists to justify the necessity of criticizing ancient medical learning. Willis begins his preface by answering an objection: what allows him to defend a new theory of fevers while "feavers have been happily cured by the same remedies, and the like method of curing, from the times of Hippocrates and Galen, even to our days"?[26] It seems to be a "rash work" to "direct his course against the received Opinion, as against a Stream."[27]

To this question, Willis responds by means of two kinds of consideration. On the one hand, we need to keep in mind that the Ancients were relying on a false position concerning the nature of diseases, because they were ignorant of the principle of blood circulation discovered by Harvey. This discovery allowed for new observations concerning the "distribution and natural motion of the nutritious humor," observations that

---

[23] However, as we will see later on, Harvey was more frequently compared to Democritus.

[24] Thomas Willis (1621–1675) was appointed Sedleian Professor of Natural Philosophy in the year 1660. See Hansruedi Isler, *Thomas Willis 1621–1675, Doctor and Scientist* (New York and London, 1968).

[25] The Latin version was published in 1659: *Diatribae duae Medico-Philosophicae quarum prior agit ... De Febribus sive de motu earumdem in sanguine animalium* (London, 1659). I quote here from the English translation, *Dr Willis Practice of Physick, Being the Whole Works* (London, 1684).

[26] What is at stake with a "new theory of feavers" is in reality a new theory of diseases. See Aubrey Davies. "Some Implications of the Circulation Theory for Disease Theory and Treatment in the 17th C," *Journal of the History of Medicine*, 26 (1971), 28-39.

[27] Thomas Willis, *The Preface to the Treatise of Feavers, Works*, "To the friendly reader," 45.

the Ancients could not make.[28] On the other hand, these new observations allowed for new experiments: the decomposition of blood into chemical principles reveals the similarity between the chemical process of fermentation (which we can observe in the production of wine or beer) and the physiological process of fever. Harvey's discovery was crucial, because it obliged those in his day to begin new enquiries concerning the nature of man and of diseases ("we ought to inquire concerning the blood").[29]

For Nedham, modern anatomical discoveries resulted in a "new frame of human nature" which rendered a "new foundation in medicine" necessary. Relying on a false conception of human nature and of nature of diseases, Hippocratism is, according to Nedham, a kind of "speculative natural philosophy." It gives rise to 'hypotheses' in the negative sense of this term: hypotheses that do not rely upon experiments and which are based on erroneous observations. "Grounded upon such doctrinal hypotheses" (such as the theory of humors), the "old medicines" are "useless" and should be replaced by "new doctrines, new methods, and rules of curation agreeable to new frame of humane nature, and to the new Phanomena of Diseases."[30]

Harvey's discovery, contrary to the ancient view, is presented by Thomas Willis in his Preface to the *Treatise of Fevers* (which is largely quoted by Nedham) as a model for thinking about the new "experimental philosophy," "characterized by a commitment to observation and experiment" and by a "very cautious application of hypotheses." While the new experimental philosophy does not prohibit the use of hypotheses, physicians should not "frame new Hypotheses to themselves from their own Ratiocination." Hypotheses should be connected to the new observations and experiments made by modern anatomists. As Willis explains, this is the only way for them to show themselves to be respectful of Hippocrates: they must give priority to observation and accept the search for new hypotheses that are able to "quadrate more exactly the Phaenomena of Feavers." As a consequence, "followers of Hippocrates" (and not Hippocrates himself) are to be blamed for the stagnation of medical art. The

---

[28] Willis, *Of Feavers, Works*, 45.
[29] *Ibid.*, 46-48.
[30] Nedham, *Medela Medicinae*, 204.

transformation of physick "into a general method" (that is to say, a speculative doctrine) is the consequence of an immoderate respect and blind veneration for the Ancients and of a lack of understanding of what is at stake in modern discoveries and experiments.[31]

It becomes urgent, therefore, to search for a new criterion to rebuild medicine on a new foundation and to define a new method of curing the sick that will take into consideration modern discoveries and new observations.

3. True and False Empiricism: Defining Empiricism as a Method

Some Considerations touching the Usefulnesse of Experimental Naturall Philosophy, The second part, Of its Usefulness to Physick was published in 1663, but it written at the end of the 1650s.[32] In the same period, Robert Boyle also stressed the fact that anatomical discoveries allow us to understand the nature of diseases better. The method used by the Ancients to deduce morbid phenomena from elementary qualities (heat, cold, humidity and dryness) must be considered as "inferiour to the Account given us of them by those ingenious Moderns, that have apply'd to the advancement of Pathologie, that Circulation of the Blood, the Motion of the Chyle by the Milky vesels to the Heart"[33] and who combined mechanical explication of the bodies ("consideration of the effects deducible from the Pores of greater bodies, and the motion and figuration of their minute parts") with "chymicall Experiments (...)."[34]

As Michael Hunter and Antonio Clericuzio have shown, Boyle does not entirely reject traditional medicine and ancient therapeutic practise.[35] He cannot, however, avoid taking position in the debate opposing defenders of traditional Galenic and Hippocratic medicine and defend-

---

31) Willis, *Of Feavers, Works*, 46.

32) Michael Hunter, *Boyle, Scrupulosity and science* (Woodbridge, 2000), ch. 8, 160.

33) Boyle refers here to John Pecquet's discovery of lymphatic system vessels, published in 1651 and translated into English in 1653: *New Anatomical Experiments of John Pecquet of Deip* (London, 1653).

34) Boyle, *Of the Usefulnesse of Naturall Philosophy* (Oxford, 1663), the second part, the first section, "Of its Usefullness to Physick," Essay II, "Offering some particulars relating to the Pathologicall Part of Physic," 28-30.

35) See Hunter, *Boyle*, 161; Clericuzio, "Les débuts," 64.

ers of the new chemical medicine. Medicine must be considered as "a Part, or an Application of natural philosophy." Following Francis Bacon's legacy, Boyle was of the opinion that the "amelioration of human life" should serve as a criterion to evaluate the usefulness of "Physic."[36] In the fifth essay of the second part of *Usefullness of Natural Philosophy*,[37] he asserts, as does Willis, that the therapeutic method (*methodus medendi*) should adapt itself to the nature of diseases revealed by modern discoveries:

> And it would be Worth an impartial disquisition, whether, since the *Methodus medendi* ought to be grounded on and accomodated to the Doctrine of Diseases, the new Anatomical discoveries formerly mention'd, and others not yet publish'd do not by innovating divers things in pathology, require some alterations & amendments in the *Methodus Mendendi*?[38]

But how should we define the aim of this new method? For Boyle, the answer is clear: "relief of the patient" should be the only criterion used to judge progress in the fields of physiology, pathology, semiotics and hygiene (that is to say, the progress accomplished in the entire practical division of medicine).[39] Boyle blames the defenders of the Hippocratic tradition for focusing on the method of observation and losing interest in the question of the cause of the disease. In the text quoted above, he mentions the case of a "witty Doctor" who preferred to give to his patient "languid remedies" instead of "more generous" ones. Because this physician blindly followed the Hippocratic method of observation he was not concerned about the death of his patient, provided that he had caused his death following the rules of the art:

> There was awhile since a witty Doctor, who being asked by an Acquaintance of mine (himself an eminent Physitian, and who related thus unto me) why he would not give such a Patient more generous remedies, seing he grew so much worse

---

36) Hunter, *Boyle*, 157.

37) Boyle, *Essay V*, 117.

38) Boyle, *Essay V*, 204.

39) Boyle, *Essay V*, 117 (emphasis added). On this division between a theoretical part and a practical part in medicine and the division of practical medicine into physiology, pathology, semiotic, hygien and therapeutic, see Harold J. Cook, "Physicians and the new Philosophy: Henry Stubbe and the virtuosi-physicians," in Roger French and Andrew Wear, eds., *The Medical Revolution of the 17th Century* (Cambridge, 1989), 247.

under the use of common languid ones, to which he had been confined, that he could not at the last but dye with them in his Mouth ? briskly answered, Let him die, if he will, so he die *secundum Artem*.[40]

But as Boyle reminds his reader, "the major part of men, who send for Physitians," are not looking to know "what ails them, as to be eas'd of it; and had not rather been methodically kill'd, then Empirically cured." What, then, is the danger of this characteristic attitude of some, but not all, physicians (as Boyle highlights)? If physicians do not care about the therapeutic effects of the method of cure, medicine will soon be given over to those "empiric physicians" already denounced by Bacon in his *Advancement of Learning* (1605), "which commonly have a few pleasing receits whereupon they are confident and adventurous, but know neither the causes of diseases, nor the complexions of patients, nor peril of accidents, nor the true methods of cures."[41] Turning the ancient medical method of observation into a speculative discourse, disconnected from therapeutic efficiency, is the best way to render medical profession "obnoxious to the cavils of such Empericks."[42]

Here is the major difficulty that defenders of medical modern discoveries have to face: the criterion of therapeutic efficiency (which serves to establish the superiority of modern medical practice over the ancient one) may be used to put into the same category defenders of "sensible experiments" in physics and "quacks" or "empericks" who are wholly ignorant of the true nature and causes of diseases and show themselves to be confident and adventurous in their use of experiments. This synonymy of "empiricism" and "charlatanism," as a kind of risky and ignorant practice of medicine, was very common during the whole of the seventeenth century. Chambers, in his *Cyclopedia*, published in London in 1728, underlines the fact, noted above, that it is used as a polemical argument by those "physicians servilely attached to the train and method of the schools, the reasonings of Hippocrates and Galen, and the statutes of the

---

[40] Boyle, *Essay* V, 118.
[41] Bacon, *The Advancement of Learning*, 10-11.
[42] "For, by such an unprofitable way of proceeding, to which some lazie, or opinionated practisers of Physick (I say some, for I mean not all), have, under pretence of its being safe, confined themselves, they have rendered their whole Profession too obnoxious to the cavils of such Empericks (...)." Boyle, *Essay* V, 118.

faculty," against "those who think more freely, and are less devoted to antiquity."[43] If the discovery of blood circulation is praised (by Willis, Boyle and later by Joseph Glanvill) for its practical and therapeutic use, defenders of Galenic method use it conversely to highlight the dangers of blood transfusion; i.e., the criterion of therapeutic efficiency may be used to invalidate the new experimental medicine as well as the ancient method of observation. This is the kind of argument that is used, for example, by Henry Stubbe in his polemic attack against defenders of modern experimental philosophy and of the emerging Royal Society, like Thomas Sprat (author of *The History of the Royal Society for the Improving of Natural Knowledge*, 1667), or Joseph Glanvill (author of *Plus Ultra: or, The Progress and advancement of knowledge since the days of Aristotle*, 1668). Whereas Stubbe warns against the danger and "ill consequences" of modern experiments, such as "injecting of Medicaments into the veins,"[44] Glanvill underlines the benefit and use of transfusion in the cure of "pleurisies, cancers, leprosies, madness, ulcers, small-pox, dotage, and all such like distempers": if "the greatest part of our Diseases arise either from the scarcity, or malignant tempers and corruptions of our blood," blood transfusion, tested by "numerous trials on several sorts of brute animals," "is an obvious remedy" and much safer than the practice of "phlebotomies" (bloodletting).[45]

Against this kind of polemical attack, according to these authors, it becomes necessary for those who want to rebuild medicine upon a new foundation to distinguish between a genuine and methodical recourse to experiment and the risky and disordered practice of quacks. On the one hand, it implies a critical attitude towards those who have turned natural philosophy into systems and discouraged men from inquiring into nature (the defenders of the Hippocratico-Galenic tradition): in-

[43] Chambers, *Cyclopeadia*, 303.
[44] Henry Stubbe, *Plus Ultra Reduced to a non plus, Of Transfusion of Blood into Animals* (London, 1670), 122. Stubbe also attacks the Royal Society in his *Legends no Histories* (London, 1670), sig. IV.
[45] Joseph Glanvill, *Plus Ultra: or, The Progress and Advancement of Knowledge since the Days of Aristotle. In an Account of Some of the most Remarkable Late Improvements of Practical, Useful Learning* (London, 1668), ch. II, 17. On this polemic between Glanvill and Stubbe, see Cook, "Physicians and the New Philosophy: Henry Stubbe and the virtuosi physicians," in French and Wear, eds., *Medical Revolution of the Seventeenth Century*, 246-71.

stead of conversing "with books" and medical authorities, instead of practising a "systematical way of writing," they should rather converse "with
things themselves."[46] On the other hand, it implies, against "empiricks"
("quacks or mountebanks"), that the search for therapeutic efficiency is
not contradictory to the search for method. Medical empiricism is not a
disordered or irrational way of inquiring into nature. Indeed, order may
proceed from careful investigation into natural phenomena and not only
from logical deduction.[47]

In other words, it is necessary to define a kind of empiricism that
would be able to "reintroduce philosophy inside medicine,"[48] a kind of
inquiry into the nature of bodies that will not give up on the investigation
into the causes of diseases. As a consequence, Boyle and others argue, it
is necessary to read again the classical texts and to search for a figure
other than Hippocrates. Such a new figure would need to be able to re-
activate this investigation into the natural characteristics of ancient empiricism even though this genuine meaning of empiricism is (following
Willis, Boyle or Nedham) now forgotten and lost.

4. Looking for a New Definition of Empiricism: Democritus versus Hippocrates

First of all, it is necessary once again to read the debate between the
empiricists and the rationalists as it is presented, for example, in Galen's
treatise *On the Sects for Beginners*. According to Galen, the empiricist and
the rationalist physician cannot understand one another. Whereas the
former declares, "I do not no know anything which goes beyond what is
apparent,"[49] the later answers that he intends to "know completely the
nature of the body he is trying to cure" and "discover causes of every

---

46) Boyle, *Certain Physiological Essays, written at distant Times, and on Several Occasions*
(London, 1661), "A Proemial Essay," 2

47) For the description of the empirical method, see Galen, *On the Sects for Beginners*,
in Richard Walzer & Michael Frede, trans. Galen, *Three Treatises on the Nature of Science*
(Indianapolis, 1985), ch. 2, 4-5.

48) Following Jackie Pigeaud, it was precisely the project of Celsus against Hippocrates
in his *De Medicina*. See Jackie Pigeaud, *Melancholia, Le malaise de l'individu* (Paris, 2008)
and *Poétiques du corps* (Paris, 2008).

49) Galen, *On the Sects*, ch. 8, 13.

disease."[50] According to the empiric sect, the knowledge of causes escapes the physician's art. We can find the same opposition in Celsus' treatise *On Medicine*. Against rationalists who pretend to know hidden causes of diseases, Celsus argues, empiricists refuse to search into remote and obscure causes, asserting that nature is incomprehensible. This is why they prohibited the practice of dissection whereas rationalists recommend it, even in the case of the vivisection of criminal bodies: it was for the rationalists the only way to discover what nature has hidden to the eyes of men.[51] Against this position defended by ancient medical empiricism, it becomes imperative for defenders of experimental philosophy, first of all, to affirm that the knowledge of nature and of natural bodies requires the use of experiments; and as far as medicine is concerned, knowledge of anatomical dissections is imperative. Secondly, they insist that the true physician must investigate the nature of the bodies he is trying to cure.

One text in particular plays a key role in working towards this reconciliation between the rationalist position and the empiric one and helps show that the search for a new explanation of diseases must be grounded upon experimentation. To those who pretend that a new doctrine of diseases or a new inquiry into the nature of man is needless, natural philosophers, like Willis or Boyle, answered quoting Celsus' words in his treatise *On Medicine*:

> It was afterwards, they proceed [*Empirici*], when the remedies has already been discovered, that men began to discuss the reasons for them: the Art of Medicine was not a discovery following upon reasoning, but after the discovery of the remedy, the reason for it was sought out.[52]

It is therefore only after remedies have been tested (some leading to recovery, others to death) that physicians are able to establish a theoretical distinction between what is beneficial and what is pernicious to health. This sentence reads like a leitmotif in the modern reading of ancient

---

[50] "The method, on the other hand, which proceeds by means of reason admonishes us to study the nature of the body which one tries to heal and the forces of all the causes which the body encounters daily." Galen, *On the Sects*, ch. 3, 5.

[51] Celsus, *De Medicina*, transl. W.G. Spencer (London, 1935), Preamble, 15.

[52] *Ibid.*, 21.

empiricism. First of all, it is used to show the necessity of an alliance between experience and reason. Medicine must be part of natural philosophy otherwise it will be surrounded by "empiricks" and "quacks." Both in his *Redargutio philosophiarum* and later in the *Novum Organum*, Bacon quotes Celsus in the same way. To remind us that "experiments" come first (collecting experimental facts and doing experiments, *historia* and *experimenta*), but only as a starting point to develop an inquiry into causes of diseases, he writes:

> And Celsus freely and wisely admits as much, namely that the experiments of medicine were invented first and only afterwards did men philosophize about them, and search out and assign the causes, and that it did not happen the other way round with the experiments themselves being discovered or produced from philosophy and knowledge of causes.[53]

Secondly, it is necessary to show that the priority given to experiments over speculative explanations implies more than a blank and passive observation of symptoms and of the development of diseases (as with the Hippocratic method).[54] Experience must have an active understanding which allows us to re-examine ancient medical doctrines. For Willis, Celsus' prescription allows for the justification of the search for a new theory of diseases and new remedies against defenders of Hippocratico-Galenic explanations of diseases who maintain that we should rely upon ancient therapeutics: "To this it will be easie to answer that Medicine was at first Empirical, and Remedies were not invented by general Precepts, but by the frequent trial of several things."[55]

However, this active meaning given to experience (experiments considered as trials or tests) implies criticism of the prohibition of dissection pronounced by Celsus. Willis and Boyle, like Bacon before them, recommend the use of comparative anatomy, which allows for the practice of

---

[53] Bacon, *Novum Organum*, I, 73, *The Oxford Francis Bacon*, Vol. XI, eds. Rees and Wakely (Oxford, 2004) 117.
[54] Bacon, *Temporis Partus Masculus*, in James Spedding, Robert Leslie Ellis and Douglas Dennon Heath, eds., *The Works of Francis Bacon* (London, 1858, repr. Stuttgart-Bad Cannstatt, 1963-94), III, 534.
[55] Willis, *Of Feavers*, "To the Reader," *Works*, 46.

dissection without the risk of being charged with inhumanity.[56] The reference to Celsus' *De Medicina* therefore usefully stressed the necessity of a "closer and purer alliance" between rationalists and empiricists. Against strict empiricism, it allowed for priority to be given to experience without giving up the inquiry into causes: medicine must be part of natural philosophy. Against dogmatic followers of the Hippocratico-Galenic method (who refused to try new remedies), it served as a reminder of the usefulness of experiments.[57]

This idea is confirmed when we turn to Boyle. In the fifth essay of *Some Considerations Touching the Usefullness of Experimental Philosophy*, he points to the fact that this judgement sentence of Celsus' could lead one to underestimate the role of reason in the discovery of therapeutic cures. And yet, it had a pedagogical function. On the one hand, those who are tempted to turn "Galenical opinion" into a system[58] must be reminded that they could, in fact, be led into neglecting useful remedies and experiments, given that they come from "illiterate people" like Paracelsus or other chemical physicians who take experiment as the only guide for medical practice. On the other hand, it must also be used against those who are tempted to forget that "experience may be uncertain without the theory of physick."[59] The "*historia facti* shall be fully and indisputably made out," and be considered as a starting point to establish new and solid "theories" which will serve "the improvement of the Therapeutical part of Physick."[60]

It is interesting to note that, according to Boyle, this dialogue between a speculative and learned form of physics and a more practical one, grounded on experimentation, may be embodied in the figure of Harvey.

---

[56] Bacon, *The Advancement of Learning*, II, 100. See also Boyle, *Of the Usefulnesse of Naturall Philosophy, Of its Usefulness to Physick, Essay I* (London, 1661), 9-10.

[57] The comparison between the "true job of the philosopher" and the activity of the bee, which "takes the middle path" between the ant ("empiricists" who "only store up and use things") and the spider ("dogmatists," who "spin webs from their own entrails") is developed in both texts some pages further than the quotation from Celsus. See for example, Bacon, *Novum Organum*, I, 95,153.

[58] Boyle, *Certain Physiological Essays, written at distant Times, and on Several Occasions*, "Proemial Essay," (London, 1661), 3.

[59] Boyle, *Some Considerations*, Essay V, ch. IX, 202. See also, Nedham, *Medela Medicinae* ch. VI, 210.

[60] Boyle, *Some Considerations*, 223-24.

It is significant that he quotes, in the same pages, Doctor Ent's "Epistle Dedicatory" to Harvey's *Anatomical Exercises on the Generation of Animals* (1651). Harvey embodies, for Boyle, the "experience'd" physician who reminds the "Learned Doctor" (George Ent, president of the Royal College of Physicians, representing the Galenic tradition and theoretical medicine) that even "barbarous nations" may discover something "for the general good, whether led to it by accident or compelled by necessity, which had been overlooked by more civilized communities."[61] Boyle uses this dialogue between Ent and Harvey to highlight the fact that physicians should not "disdain the Remedies of such illiterate People, only because of their being unacquainted with our Theory of Physick."[62] Later on, he explains how Harvey, "as rigid a Naturalist he is, scrupled not to try the Experiment mentioned by Helmont"; that is to say, magnetic cures or cures "by transplantation."[63] Harvey embodies a figure of the physician able to reconcile the use of experiments (coming from chemical medicine, and especially from Helmontianism) with an active inquiry into the nature of phenomena. Besides, we should not forget the comparison developed in Ent's "Epistle Dedicatory" between Harvey and Democritus, the ancient philosopher known to be a untiring investigator of nature. Ent reports a conversation between Harvey and himself at the end of the 1640's when the famous English physician retires and takes shelter in his brother's house in Surrey, far away from the troubles of the civil war: "I found him Democritus like, busy with the study of natural things," writes Ent.[64]

This picture of Harvey as a new Democritus is commonplace in the English natural philosophical literature during the 1650s. Walter Charleton, the eclectic physician close to chemical medicine who was also a defender of corpuscular explanations of natural phenomena calls Harvey "our Democritus Londinensis."[65] This comparison is useful in defending

---

61) "Doctor Ent's Epistle Dedicatory," *Anatomical Exercises on the Generation of Animals*, in Willis, ed., *The Works of William Harvey* (London, 1847), 146-47.
62) Boyle, *Some Considerations*, 223.
63) *Ibid.*, 231.
64) "Doctor Ent's Epistle Dedicatory," 145.
65) Walter Charleton, *Physiologia Epicuro-Gassendo-Charltoniana, or a Fabrik of Science Natural, Upon the Hypothesis of Atoms. Founded by Epicurus, Repaired by Petrus*

Harvey's discoveries and for recommending an active investigation into nature and the use of dissection.[66]

In the fourth essay of the first part of the *Usefulnesse of Experimental Naturall Philosophy* (written in the mid-1650s), Boyle shows himself to be quite critical of modern followers of the ancient atomists (Lucretian atomism), who try to "exclude deity from intermeddling with matter" and think of matter as something active. Against this possible atheistic use of atomism, Boyle stresses how the decomposition of the body into its minute parts allows the atomist to admire "the omniscient Author of Nature."[67] Later on, in *The Excellency of Theology compar'd with Natural Philosophy* (1674), Boyle returns to this "modest and useful way practis'd by the Antients [and especially by Democritus] of inquiring into particular bodies, without hastening to make systems," which was recently restored by "two of our London Physicians, Gilbert and Harvey."[68] If modern discoveries about the power of magnets or the blood circulation must be praised, it is because they renew the atomistic or corpuscular approach[69] practised by Democritus as well as Leucippus, Epicurus and "almost all the Naturalists that preceded Aristotle."[70] Against Aristotelian and Galenic followers, who still urge one to "deduce the Pheanomena

---

Gassendus, Augmented by Walter Charleton (London, 1654). Charleton, *Darkness of Atheism* (London, 1651), 130-31.

[66] See for example how it is used by Zacharie Wood (Sylvius) in the preface to the first Dutch edition of the *De Motu Cordis*. *The Anatomical Exercises of Dr. William Harvey* (...) *with The Preface of Zachariah Wood, Physician of Rotterdam* (London, 1653).

[67] "And certainly, he that shall see a skilfull Anatomist dextrously dissect that admirable part of Man, the Eye, and shall consider the curious contrivance of the several coats, humors and other parts it consists of, with all their adaptations and uses, would be easily perswaded, That a good Anatomist has much stronger Invitations to believe, and admire an Omnicient Anthor of Nature, than he that never saw a Dissection (...)." Boyle, *Usefullnesse of Experimental Naturall Philosophy* (Oxford, 1663) Essay IV, 95.

[68] William Gilbert (1540–1603), a physician known for his research on the power of magnets.

[69] Renewed by the work of Peter Gassendi. On this praise of Gassendi for having resurrected: "the atomism of Democritus, Leucippus, and Epicurus, after it had been long submerged by the Peripateticke Philosophy," see Royal Society, Boyle Papers, "Of Atoms," quoted by Robert G. Franck, *Harvey and the Oxford Physiologists* (Berkeley, Los Angeles and London, 1980), 94.

[70] Boyle, *The Excellency of Theology Compared with Natural Philosophy* (London, 1674), 199.

from the four qualities, the four elements, and some few other barren hypotheses, ascribing what could not be explicated by them (...) to substantial Forms and occult qualities,"[71] it is necessary to come back to this active and careful investigation of natural phenomena which only try to explain things in terms of "Bigness, shape, motion, &c. of corpuscules, or the minutest active parts of Matter."[72] Democritus, known for his "particular experiments and observations" and for his "manifold dissections of Animals" appears here again as a key figure in the defence of the idea that this active observation of natural phenomena is the only way to clear natural philosophy and especially medicine of the "barren hypotheses" or "narrow principles" of the "Peripateticks."

We are now able to grasp the double function of the comparison between Democritus and Harvey, between the careful and scrupulous observation of particular bodies and the experimental method grounded upon a corpuscular approach to natural bodies. On the one hand, it serves to build an alternative model for the investigation of nature. Physicians should rely not upon the passive observation of symptoms, like Hippocrates proposed, but should act like Democritus, who was not afraid of making "anatomical dissections of living animals." Boyle explains, in a *Letter to Frederik Clod*, that he was convinced by Harvey's discovery of blood circulation, not by reading books but by engaging with the practice of dissection under the assistance of William Petty.[73] On the other hand, this comparison is also useful in explaining the rejection of the new "corpuscularian philosophy" and, more generally, of "experimen-

---

71) Boyle, *The Excellency*, 200.

72) *Ibid.*, 199.

73) "For my part, that I may not live wholly useless, or altogether a stranger in the study of nature, since I want glasses and furnaces to make a chemical analysis of inanimate bodies, I am exercising myself in making anatomical dissections of living animals: wherein (being assisted by your father-in-law's ingenious friend Dr. Petty, our general's physician) I have satisfied myself of the circulation of the blood, and the (freshly discovered and hardly discoverable) receptacumul chyli, made by the confluence of the venae lacteae; and have seen (especially in the dissections of fishes) more of the variety and contrivances of nature, and the majesty and wisdom of her author, than all the books I ever read in my life could five me convincing notions of." Boyle to Frederick Clod, in Boyle, *Works*, ed., Birch, vol VI (Hildesheim, 1966), 54-55.

tal philosophy."[74] Like Democritus, Harvey had to face the incomprehension of his contemporaries. We should not forget how Democritus is pictured in the *Pseudo-Hippocratic Letters*.[75] Devoting all his time to the dissection of beasts he is reputed by his fellow Abderites to have been mad. But the eventual meeting between the allegedly mad philosopher and the great physician Hippocrates, called in to cure him, reveals that truth can only result from this precise dissection of nature. Democritus, then, was the perfect figure for justifying the necessity of experimenting upon animal bodies and thus of engaging in comparative anatomy.

When Glanvill, in his *Plus Ultra* (1668), highlights those arts that may increase knowledge, he refers largely to anatomy. Democritus is praised again for having cleared medicine of the charge of being inhuman in dissecting bodies, showing that it was possible to practice it upon animals. Democritus "was fain to excuse his dissection of Beasts, even to the great Hippocrates."[76] He is a key figure to establish the superiority of "experimental philosophy" against "speculative natural philosophy."[77] In the meantime, referring to this ancient figure of the natural philosopher is useful also in explaining the violence of the critics and the accusations levelled at the modern pioneers; especially in the case of those who, like Harvey, used their "wit and industry" to investigate and reveal a new "Oeconomy of human Nature," which differed greatly from the Hippocratic view of human nature.

5. Conclusion

By way of conclusion, I would like to stress why it is necessary to study medical debates if we want to understand the genesis and nature of mod-

---

[74] See Boyle, *The Excellency*, 200-201. On the critique of experimental philosophy, see for example Michael Hunter, *Establishing the New Science. The Experience of the Early Royal Society* (New York, 1989) and also Rosemary H. Syfret, "Some Early Critics of the Royal Society," *Notes and Records of the Royal Society of London*, 8.1 (London, 1950), 20-64.

[75] Hippocrates, *Pseudepigraphic Writings, Letters—Embassy—Speech from the Alter—Decree*, transl. Wesley D. Smith (Leiden, New York and Cologne, 1990), 49-109.

[76] Glanvill, *Plus Ultra*, 13.

[77] Anstey, "Experimental versus Speculative Natural Philosophy," in Peter Anstey & John A. Schuster, eds., *The Science of Nature in Seventeenth Century. Patterns of Change in Early Natural Philosophy* (Dordrecht, 2005), 215-42.

ern philosophical empiricism. As I have tried to demonstrate, the question here is whether modern medical discoveries (blood circulation, lymphatic system, new theory of fevers) engage with a "new frame of human nature." This argument plays a key role in justifying new methods of investigating the causes of diseases and defining new ways of curing human bodies. It is this motive that moves modern philosophers to return to the classical medical tradition and to deal with the old debates around the true method (*medendus medendi*). As we have seen, however, there are different ways of reading the tradition of ancient empiricism. If Hippocrates must be praised for having given attention to empirical observation, there is also an urgent need to define more active ways of investigating natural bodies. Democritus appears here as a counterweight to define empiricism as a true method (against "empiricks" or "quacks") and to show that giving priority to experience does not lead to giving up the search for causes, even if we may merely grasp probable causes without any claim to certain knowledge about the nature of man and of disease.

If we want to overcome the vagueness of the label of 'empiricism' (too often opposed to 'rationalism' in a caricatured way), we must pay attention to the various meanings this word has had in the field of medical knowledge and to the different figures who were used to defend a practical philosophical approach against a speculative one. Medicine and not physics alone plays a great role in this story. Taking into consideration its very controversial nature in the middle of the seventeenth century has allowed us to show the presence of two distinct anti-speculative traditions (the phenomenalist tradition following Hippocrates and the experimentalist one following Democritus) in the genesis of modern philosophical empiricism.

The Status of Leibniz' Medical Experiments:
A Provisional Empiricism?

Anne-Lise Rey

*Université Lille I/UMR Savoirs, Textes, Langage**

Abstract

This paper examines the status of medical experiments using the Leibnizian conception of knowledge. The aim is to consider whether experimentation is a "perceptive foretaste" or a real condition for the advancement of knowledge. To this end I argue, first, that acting on bodies could be a way to understand them and, second, I establish a place for medical experiments in the field of learning. In these ways, I identify a "provisional empiricism" in Leibniz' medical texts.

Keywords

G.W. Leibniz, medicine, experiments, empiricism, knowledge

It is difficult, though tempting, to consider Leibniz' approach to the body as perfectly autonomous, governed by the metaphysical considerations regarding the machine of nature and the "invention" of the notion of the organism, and at the same time by his unfailingly vivid interest in medical practice (medical remedies, projects for listing symptoms, diseases, climatic conditions, the efficacy of medicines, and so on).[1] Should this

---

* Université Lille I, Cité scientifique, 59655 Villeneuve d'Ascq Cedex, France (annelise. rey@free.fr).

[1] This paper was translated by Marjorie Sweetko and linguistically improved by Thomas Swan. I would like to thank Justin Smith for his careful reading of this article. For Leibniz and the machine of nature, see Michel Fichant, "Leibniz et les machines de la nature," *Studia Leibnitiana*, 35 (1) (2003), 1-28. Justin E. H. Smith and Ohad Nachtomy, eds., *Machines of Nature and Corporeal Substances in Leibniz* (Dordrecht, 2011);. Pauline Phemister, *Leibniz and the Natural World: Activity, Passivity and Corporeal Substances in Leibniz' Philosophy* (Dordrecht, 2005); Enrico Pasini, *Corpo e funzioni cognitive in Leibniz*, "Pubblicazioni del 'Centro di studi del pensiero filosofico del Cinquecento e del Seicento

disparate collection of works be taken simply as more proof of Leibniz'
extraordinary curiosity regarding what he calls "the most necessary of
the natural sciences?"[2] Nothing could be less certain! Rather than contrasting a rational medicine, the clearest expression of which was to be
found in the work of Friedrich Hoffman (who is supposed to have taken
medicine a step closer to fitting with the theory of the monad), with a
practical medicine satisfied with producing fragmentary and inconclu-
sive lists, our aim here is to elucidate the status and the role of experiments in Leibniz' medical thought.[3] In so doing, I aim to distinguish

---

in relazione ai problemi della scienza' del CNR" (Milan, 1996), 238; François Duchesneau,
Leibniz, le vivant et l'organisme (Paris, 2010); and Justin E. H. Smith, *Divine Machines*
(Princeton, 2010). For Leibniz and the notion of organism, see Raphaële Andrault, who
clearly showed how this notion takes shape in Leibniz' writings through a dialogue with
Nehemiah Grew, which was typical of the physico-theological interpretations of the
organism current at the turn of the eighteenth century. See "Entre anatomie et théolo-
gie: l'organisme chez Nehemiah Grew et G.W. Leibniz," *Natur und Subjekt. IX. Internationaler Leibniz-Kongress*, ed. Herbert Breger, Jürgen Herbst and Sven Erdner (Hannover,
2011), I, 18-26. Examples of Leibniz' interest in medicine are: "Secrets médicinaux con-
sidérables et pour la pluspart épouvez tirez d'un livre in 8° écrit de la main de feu Mons.
Acar, homme tres erudit et qui faisait des experiences (Ms, LBr III, IV, 8a Bl.1)," or
"Essence styptique qui arrête le sang, inventée par M. de la Rivière" (Ms, LH III, 5, Bl
86-87), and of course "Excerptum ex Autographo Cartesii" (Ms, LH III, 5, 49 et seq).
There are, therefore, a number of short texts, rarely referred to, which would appear to
indicate more than a simple curiosity in medical matters on Leibniz' part.

[2]   Letter from Leibniz to Fr. Bouvet, 1697, entitled: "Des Cartésiens: De la philosophie
pratique: De la Physique, et de la Médecine"), in Leibniz, *Opera omnia*, ed. Louis Dutens
(Geneva, 1768), II, 1, 262-63.

[3]   As for Friedrich Hoffman, he was a German physician and chemist from Halle (1662-
1740) was the author of *Medicina rationalist sytematica* in 6 volumes, published in 6
volumes in Halle between 1718 and 1734. He considereds the human body to be a hydraulic machine entirely governed by mechanical laws. François Duchesneau shows well
in *Leibniz, le vivant et l'organisme* (Paris, 2010), how Leibniz' support for Hoffman's
rational medicine is accompanied by an obvious desire to make room for the concrete
lessons which the senses can teach us. (p. 158). Grmek displays in his article on how
Leibniz considers mercury, sulfur and salt as powers or levels of activity, and mobilizes
what he calls a "rational therapeutics." Here, the practice is understood as the presence
of an active principle in matter and more specifically of a level of activity. (Cf. Grmek,
Mirko Drazen Grmek, "Leibniz et la médecine pratique," in Grmek, *Leibniz 1646-1716.
Aspects de l'homme et de l'oeuvre* (Paris, 1968), 145-77). On Leibniz' view of practical
medicine, see Leibniz' Letter to Nicolas Hartsoeker of 12 December 1706, *Die philosophischen Schriften von G.W. Leibniz* ed. C.J. Gerhardt (Berlin, 1875-1890; repr. Hildesheim,

between the indispensable use of experimentation in establishing medical knowledge and a "provisional empiricism," covering at the same time both the extreme fecundity of experimentation in terms of knowledge and its double function of providing a rough foretaste of knowledge to come.[4] This article will be devoted to outlining these two aspects of experimentation, and to establishing the criteria required to distinguish between them.

To this end, it is useful to remember what Leibniz said to Christiaan Huygens in his letter of the 2nd of May, 1691: "I prefer a Leeuwenhoek who tells me what he sees to a Cartesian who tells me what he thinks."[5] I intend to explore the reasons for this preference from two viewpoints, examining the various ways in which the question of visibility affects medical knowledge; or to put it another way, it seems to me that this reference to "a Leeuwenhoek who tells me what he sees" shows that Leibniz is reflecting on the new conditions of the visibility of the body obtained via the microscope, in what constitutes a new visual acuity.[6] This was due to a change in attitude toward the function of anatomy—a new approach to exploring the body—and to the importance and meaning that was to be given to the constitution of *anatomical analysis*.[7] This

---

1965) (henceforth *GP*), vol. III, 489. On the role of experiments in Leibniz' thought, see Johannes Steudel's book, *Leibniz und die Medizin* (Bonn, 1960) and Fritz Hartmann's works on medicine and Leibniz in his report of the theory of knowledge, which played a pioneering role. Cf. for example, Fritz Hartmann and Matthias Krüger, "Methoden ärztlicher Wissenschaft bei Leibniz," in *Akten des 2. Internationalen Leibniz-Kongresses, Hannover, 17.-22. Juli 1972* (Wiesbaden, 1973), 1, 235-47 and mainly the famous Hartmann and Krüger, "Directiones ad rem medicam pertinentes. Ein Manuskript G.W. Leibnizens aus den Jahren 1671/72 über die Medizin," *Studia Leibnitiana*, 8 (1976) 40-68.

[4] This idea of a "provisional empiricism" is certainly related to seventeenth-century Galenism. François Duchesneau, *La physiologie des Lumières, Archives internationales d'histoire des idées* (The Hague, Boston and London, 1982), in chapter III devoted to Leibniz and entitled "Critique et synthèse leibniziennes," 80, writes: "Or, ce que l'on ignore généralement et dont il faut tenir compte c'est la "ruse" leibnizienne qui consistait à promouvoir une forme d'empirisme préliminaire et à se défier des spéculations métaphysiques dans les travaux de physiologie et de médecine."

[5] Letter to Christiaan Huygens, in *Œuvres completes de Christiaan Huygens*, ed. Hollandsche Maatschappij der Wetenschappen, X (The Hague, 1905), 52.

[6] On this relationship, see Gennar Luigi Linguiti, *Leibniz e la scoperta del mondo microscopico della vita* (Lucca, 1984).

[7] Cf. the change in attitude to the anatomy at the turn of the 18th eighteenth century.

resulted in fact in an awareness of the fruitful lessons that can be drawn from comparative anatomy understood as a "microscope of nature."[8] It is thus worth pointing out their impact on the reconfiguration of medical knowledge, as well as on the manner in which this "new way of looking," this "mutation of the visible," has led towards a re-examination of the epistemological palette that takes us from hypothesis to factual certainty.[9]

Acting on the Bodies, so as to Know them?

Elsewhere, I have described the central importance of the ambivalent notion of action (*actio in se ipsum*) in understanding the internal force at work in physical bodies as a sign of substantiality.[10] François Duchesneau has established how very fruitful it was to use such dynamics in understanding organic bodies.[11] One principal question arises in this respect: does acting on the body enable us to understand its inner workings? How, in other words, can the true weight Leibniz' philosophy affords to observation and experimentation in the search for knowledge of the body be assessed? Can they in fact be turned into epistemological modalities? I intend here to determine the weight that Leibniz gives to

---

Rafael R. Mandressi has pointed out clearly how anatomy constructs a body and the important role played by analysis in this construction. Rafael Mandresi, *Le regard de l'anatomiste, Dissections et invention du corps en Occident* (Paris, Seuil, 2003), 16.

[8] François Duchesneau refers in *Les modèles du vivant de Descartes à Leibniz* to Luigi Belloni, who in his introduction to the works of Marcello Malpighi mentions the *Exercitatio anatomico-medica de glandulis in intestino duodeno hominis detectis* (Heidelberg, 1687), 12. As stated by Mandressi, "ce traité prône le remplacement de la simple dissection par la *resolutio ad minutum*." Mandressi, *Le regard de l'anatomiste*, 148.

[9] To use Philippe Hamou's evocative title, *La mutation du visible. Essai sur la portée épistémologique des instruments d'optique au XVIIème siècle* (Villeneuve d'Ascq, 2001).

[10] Following on from the work of Michel Fichant and the article "De la puissance à l'action: la singularité stylistique de la dynamique " in Fichant, *Science et métaphysique dans Descartes et Leibniz* (Paris, 1995), 205-43. In two separate articles, I have shown the importance of this ambivalence. Cf. "L'ambivalence de la notion d'action dans la Dynamique de Leibniz: la correspondance entre Leibniz et De Volder," I, *Studia Leibnitiana*, 41 (2009), 47-66 and II, *Studia Leibnitiana*, 41 (2011), 157-82.

[11] Duchesneau, *Leibniz, le vivant et l'organisme*, esp. ch. 3, "Les machines leibniziennes de la nature," 93 ff.

experiments in the constitution of a body of knowledge in the natural sciences. Thus, I begin by placing the heuristic practice of intervention on the body, specific to medicine, within the general framework of the principles of the intelligibility of nature set down by Leibniz, linking it to the status of observation, a status newly upgraded in recognition of the significant advances made possible by the use of the microscope.

Leibniz clearly makes a distinction between observation and experimentation, but he nevertheless includes them both under the same heading of that which is "inductive," leading to perceptible truths.[12]

Medical Observation

In the 1670s, Leibniz praised the microscope as a way of expanding the boundaries of the visible and, thus, of the knowable. How seeing leads to knowing is described several times over by Leibniz, most often under Hooke's influence. At the same time, Leibniz explains in practical terms how to build a microscope, and how large numbers of them can open the way to a "theatre of nature" consisting of a "whole cabinet of microscopes" which will lead to rapid progress.[13]

Here he is subscribing to a movement which has been admirably explored by Catherine Wilson, Christoph Lüthy and Philippe Hamou, who to varying degrees underline the speculative use of the microscope.[14] As Hamou documents, in the first half of the seventeenth century "what the

---

[12] This will be subsequently seen in *Veritates physicae*, in *Gottfried Wilhelm Leibniz: Sämtliche Schriften und Briefe*, ed. Deutsche Akademie der Wissenschaften zu Berlin (Darmstadt, Leipzig, Berlin, Akademie-Verlag, 1992-2010) (henceforth *A*), VI, 4, where Leibniz clearly states that inductions are universal objective truths in agreement with a great number of individual truths. They are either observations or experiments.

[13] Cf. for example Leibniz' letter to Jean-Paul de la Roque at the end of 1677 (A, III, 2, 259-262).

[14] Catherine Wilson, *The Invisible World. Early Modern Philosophy and the Invention of the Microscope* (Princeton, 1995). Christoph Lüthy shows in particular the close link between the successful introduction of the microscope and the procedures to institute corpuscular theories in the seventeenth century in his unpublished thesis "Matter and Microscopes in the Seventeenth Century" (PhD thesis, Harvard University, 1995). Hamou, *La mutation*, 2, 104, explains how the microscope opened the way to "l'espoir nouveau d'une visualisation des constituants premiers de la matière."

instrument shows people has less impact than what it suggests to them."[15] The originality of Hooke's *Micrographia* of 1665 resides, still according to Hamou, "in the objective, which it manifests and which it achieves, of reconciling the visible and the speculative: for the first time, the philo-sophical intentions connected with microscopy (the mechanistic and corpuscular hypothesis) will be seriously attached to the concrete visibil-ity offered by the instrument."[16] In other words, if it was true that the new visibility offered by the microscope guaranteed access to the intelligibil-ity of non-visible things, then this, at least in Hooke's work, was linked to a concern, not devoid of ambiguities (as pointed out by Lüthy), that they should fit into the mechanical framework of a "real alphabet."[17]

This, then, is our challenge: Should Leibniz' enthusiasm for the use of the microscope in medicine be viewed from the perspective of the frame-work of intelligibility involved in his project for a universal characteris-tic? In this case, we would need to understand exactly how this new visibility is construed by Leibnitz as a legitimate procedure for under-standing the living body. Is he trying, as with Hooke (whom he regularly cites) or Leeuwenhoek (whom he frequently praises), to make it a new universal organ; or on the contrary, to limit its use to a few specific fields of learning without proclaiming the need for a profound change in the systems of intelligibility involved in natural philosophy based on these new ways of seeing?

The beginnings of a reply to this question can be found in a text en-titled *Directiones ad rem medicam pertinentes*.[18] The text in fact opens with a reminder of the importance of research on urine and the pulse. To prove this importance, Leibniz states: "We must have instruments to do specific research on urine and the pulse, for they are generally indica-

---

[15] Hamou, *La mutation*, 115-16.

[16] *Ibid.*, 117. See also *ibid.*, 124-25, still regarding Hooke: The microscope would allow us access to "les mécanismes infimes qui permettront d'expliquer les qualités apparentes non plus hypothétiquement, mais dans le cadre d'une philosophie "réelle," fondée sur une expérience authentique."

[17] See in particular, Christoph Lüthy, "Atomism, Lynceus, and the Fate of Seventeenth-Century Microscopy," *Early Science and Medicine*, 1 (1996), 1-27.

[18] LH III, 1, 3, folio 1-9. This text was critically examined by Hartmann and Krüger, *Studia Leibnitiana, Sonderheft*, 8 (1971), 40-68. An English translation appears in Appen-dix I of Smith, *Divine Machines*, 277-89.

tors *of the human condition.*"[19] He continues: "For urine, there is nothing better than a good microscope with one objective, for this will reveal thousands of things that cannot otherwise be found in urine and will quickly engender rules far superior to all those previously in use." Other examples of observations are contained in the same text: of the pulse, of the warmth and coldness of the hands, etc. While the microscope is clearly shown to be useful for the analysis of urine as a way to learn about and treat the body, it is not alone in this and is accompanied by other analytical practices borrowed explicitly from chemical medicine: the text shows that Leibniz also considers it important to weigh, distil or clarify urine and blood.[20]

Thus, observation is considered one of the practices that can lead to a better understanding of those invisible constituents of the human body that explain its disturbances. I use this example to show that Leibniz clearly places his reflection within the framework of the Royal Society's research on *experimental philosophy* and that he fully endorses the idea that microscopic observation is crucial in *anatomical analyses,* going so far as to conceive of it as a decisive instrument for attaining knowledge of the human body.

Medical Experimentation

The term *medical experimentation* is used here to mean acting on the bodies with a view not only to treating them but also, and perhaps principally, to learning about them. So while the purpose of this action on the bodies is to reveal the nature of the natural processes, it necessarily involves the modalities by which the process is grasped and, therefore, needs to be linked to a method of interpreting something which, in passing from the invisible to the visible, has become a sign.

Intervention on the body may be very explicit; for example, Leibniz suggests having an individual ingest emetics in order to elucidate the process by which the *action* of vomiting occurs. Here, it is through the

---

[19] I quote from the English translation: "One must have instruments for precisely investigating the urine and the pulse, since these are generally signs of a man's condition," Smith, *Divine Machines,* 277.

[20] Smith, *Divine Machines,* 278.

artificial reproduction of a natural process that learning and understanding are achieved.

As Justin Smith has shown, Leibniz' interest in emetics continues at least until the publication of his treatise *De novo antidysenterico* in 1695-6, devoted to *ipecacuanha*.[21] The metaphysical issue behind this interest is illustrated by Smith in the first chapter of *Divine Machines*:

> Leibniz is interested not just in the pathology of vomiting, but also in inducing vomiting experimentally in order to see what the food is doing in the stomach. [...] Leibniz shares in the commonplace view that digestion, the transformation of food into flesh, is, as Walter Charleton would put it, "nothing else but Generation continued" to the extent that many of the same physical processes must take place in the one case as in the other, and to the extent that at a metaphysical level both involve the transformation of aggregate matter into corporeal-substance matter.[22]

Smith also comments on this interest ("Leibniz' call for the experimental use"), comparing it to the way in which Harvey observes the different stages of development of the foetus; he describes it as a new way of getting inside a natural process (nutrition or generation) which is usually hidden. In setting up this veritable experimental protocol (actually causing a natural process to occur artificially in order to understand it), Leibniz was integrating into his epistemological horizon the importance of the intervention on the body as a cognitive modality.

Having given various examples of Leibniz' interest in these heuristic practices, I will now use a relatively well-known passage from Leibniz' correspondence to situate them in the context of the overall search for knowledge of nature, so as to shed light on the special status he affords to medical observation and experimentation.

The Construction of Medical Observation and Experimentation as Distinct Epistemological Modalities

Numerous texts testify to Leibniz' commitment to a heuristic use of microscopic observation and experimentation in medicine, but the central

---

[21] Leibniz, "Relatio ad Inclytam Societatem Leopoldinam Nat. Curios. de Novo Anti-dysenterico Americano, magnis successibus comprobato," *Journal de Leipzig* (December 1695), 559.

[22] *Ibid.*, 34.

question pertains to the function he gives them within his epistemological economy: should the recurring references to the advances made
via the use of microscopes, the praises heaped on Leeuwenhoek in a
range of texts published in learned journals and the importance given to
bodily experimentation in medicine be taken as mere awareness by Leibniz of the "experimental philosophy" of his time, such as it was developing around the Royal Society? Of course they should. Should these
cognitive practices be seen, above all, as undervalued by the critical literature precisely because they rely heavily on the world of experience?
I believe so. Nevertheless, as Smith says in the opening words of the first
chapter of *Divine Machines:* "We do not tend to think today of medicine
as a foundational science, let alone as an important component of
philosophy."[23] My intention here is not to reveal the central but hidden
dimension that medicine assumes in philosophy, but rather to demonstrate that Leibniz' reflections on experiments, if examined with rigor,
can shed light on the Leibnizian philosophical reflection on the body and
the place of experimentation in his epistemology.

In a letter of the 26th of May, 1714 to Abbé Jean-Paul Bignon, counsel-
lor to the king and president of the Royal Academy of Sciences, Leibniz
reflects on how to further scientific progress:

> I would wish that greater attention were given to advances in practical Medicine,
> by distinguishing the simple hypothesis from the plausible conjecture, and the very
> likely conjecture from the factual certainty. But above all, that more attention were
> paid to making and recording observations; and I would like any Physician who
> discovers a new practical aphorism, ordinarily true and found through observation,
> to be rewarded.[24]

Of course, this letter comes late in Leibniz' life, being written two years
before his death, but it reflects in its own way on his emphasis on observation and perhaps most important on the cleavage that occurs in the
writings of Leibniz between the texts of the 1670s, primarily the *Directiones* of 1671, which give a central place to the intervention on the body and
to animal experimentation, and the texts of the 1680s, which emphasize

---

[23] Smith, *Divine Machines,* 25.
[24] Marc Amsler "Une lettre de Leibniz. Transcription et notes," *Gesnerus,* 19 (1962),
37-38.

pure observation. As is clearly shown by Smith, this epistemological difference can be explained by a change in the models of the body, explaining what the animal machine is: we move from a hydraulic-pneumatic
model to an organic model in the specific sense that Leibniz assigns to
it. It is through this cleavage, furthermore, that we must understand observation and experimentation not only as two distinct epistemological
terms but also as two distinct moments in the constitution of Leibnizian
epistemology.

From the multitude of passages on the status of medical practice, I
have chosen the passage quoted above in particular because it seems to
me that it explicitly defines what Leibniz considers the central issues in
medical experimentation. First, it gives value to the collecting of observations within practical medicine. Indeed, this is one of the projects Leibniz constructs around the political need to organize the collection of
symptoms and effective treatments in the interests of the advancement
of our knowledge.[25] This promotion of observation should be seen in the
context of the new opportunities for observation offered by the microscope, which explains the recurring references to Leeuwenhoek. Second,
it establishes a link between this valuing of observation and the level of
plausibility of the knowledge acquired. In the passage quoted above, by
proposing hierarchical distinctions between hypothesis, plausible conjecture, very likely conjecture and factual certainty, Leibniz clearly links
practical medicine and conjecture.

Leibniz treated the status of this conjectural knowledge in his *Praefatio ad Libellum Elementorum Physicae*[26] After recognizing that the most
perfect method consists in finding the inner constitution of the bodies a

---

[25] Cf., for example, Leibniz, "Extrait d'une lettre sur la manière de perfectionner la
médecine," *Journal des Sçavans* (July 1694), in *Opera omnia*, ed. Dutens, II, 2, 162-63,
where he refers to the project of creating a history of medicine in Paris, similar to that
created by Bernardino Ramazzini.

[26] This commitment to conjecture is found in the 13th doubt addressed to Stahl (Sarah
Carvallo, *Stahl-Leibniz: la controverse sur la vie, l'organisme et le mixte* (Paris, 2004), 91.
For the *Praefatio ad Libellum Elementorum Physicae*, see Leibniz, *A*, VI, 4. Duchesneau
has admirably analyzed this text, in particular highlighting "les modes de transition
entre la connaissance empirique et la science rationnelle des phénomènes organiques"
in chapter II of *Leibniz, le vivant et l'organisme*, in a chapter entitled "Leibniz et le des-
sein d'une science des vivants," 66-70, esp. 68.

priori—that is, starting from the contemplation of the author of things—
he immediately adds that this is very difficult.[27] This is why he proposes
to distinguish between two methods of reasoning from experiments, one
for the use and the other for the cause.[28] This method of finding the
causes is itself double : one is a priori and certain, the other is *a posteriori* and conjectural. In recognizing that this manner of finding the causes
is not easily accessible, however, Leibniz is led to expand on this method
of reasoning from experiments to find causes, and he explains that it
presupposes that phenomena can be determined through their attributes.

This text indicates at the same time three separate points. The first is
that there is a veritable experimental terrain within which the analytical
break-down of phenomena into their primary constituents enables the
causes of the phenomena to be identified. It thus becomes possible to
break with the traditional distinction between a practical medicine that
treats symptoms and a rational medicine that identifies the causes and
that shows that by starting from experience and conducting a rigorous
analysis, it is possible to identify the cause of diseases. The second is that
when it is impossible, as with medical diagnosis, to decide among several possible causes, the true cause introduces a process of selection and
elimination of possible causes; for example, diseases. The third and final
point is that this means of selection is considered probable.

It seems to me that this sort of 'reverse engineering' from experiments
to causes clearly reveals a project for a 'medical characteristic' (if I may)
which would provide medicine with a reference point from which to
assess the reliability and the degree of certainty of the knowledge acquired through these experiments.[29]

Leibniz did produce a short text that somewhat clarifies this link between medical experiments and the certainty of knowledge, which
should be located in the wider context of what Leibniz calls physical
truths. This could be seen as natural enough, since Leibniz explicitly
describes medicine as a special type of physics. In this text, dating from

---

[27] Leibniz, *Praefatio*, A, VI, 4, 1998.
[28] *Ibid.*, A, VI, 4, 1995.
[29] *Ibid.*, A, VI, 4, 1999.

1678 or 1680 and entitled *Veritates physicae,* Leibniz distinguishes three types of physical truth: intellectual, sensible (*sensuales*) and mixed.[30] The physical truths which are sensible (*sensuales*) are those that we discover through the senses alone and they are either histories or inductions. Histories are individual sensible truths, like the relationship of the eclipse with a lunar feature. Inductions, on the other hand, are universal sensible truths in agreement with a large number of individual truths and are either observations or experiments (*experimenta*). Thus, Leibniz distinguishes observations as being inductions requiring us to act as spectators and experiments as being inductions where we touch bodies or even modify them, as in the case of chemical experiments. Inductions have degrees of universality, and some are more certain than others. Leibniz provides the example: no sensible person can doubt that the sun will rise tomorrow but that rhubarb is a purgative cannot be asserted with the same certainty. Yet this text introduces a significant variant: it opens with Leibniz proposing a distinction between different physical truths: not between the intellectual and the sensible but between the dogmatic and the empirical. Defining empirical truths as those proven through the experience of the senses, either as experiments (*experimenta*) or as observations.

This text is important because it shows that Leibniz is thinking specifically about medical experimentation within the framework of a notion of sensible truth achieved by induction, which involves acting on the body, and whose degree of certainty is variable, being relative to individual reaction. He is advancing here the idea of universal sensible truths; a kind of universality obtained through induction. This touches on the central idea that I am presenting here: the idea of a *provisional empiricism*. The knowledge achieved is provisional to the extent that it is conceived of as awaiting corroboration or rectification by rational knowledge. In fact, in a totally different context, Leibniz states that the universals based on induction are never perfectly certain until we know the reason behind them.[31] Nevertheless, I believe that Leibniz, through the roles that he assigns to them, is granting medical observation and experimentation the status of fully-fledged epistemological modalities:

---

[30] *Ibid., A,* VI, 4, 1983-85.
[31] "Extrait du dictionnaire de M. Bayle, article Rorarius p.2599 sqq.de l'édition de l'an 1702 avec mes remarques." (*GP* IV, 526).

their very shortcomings on symptoms or the unreliability of remedies enable us to discover the true nature of bodies.

The "Experimental Principles": Legitimizing Medical Experiments?

In this paper, I intend to show that, when Leibniz places this value on medical experimentation in his cognitive system, there is always a parallel attack on these heuristic practices on the grounds of their "excessive" empiricity. This is particularly evident in the *Replicationes* to Stahl (especially Reply XI), which lay down the conditions for legitimate medical experiment. It is important to note from the outset that Leibniz uses the term 'empirical' in a wide sense: whenever he gives the reasons for these empirical failings, he states that he is referring to discussions of the human body which are based on observations. I am thinking in particular of the opening lines of Reply XI (3rd point):

> I have often pointed out that Medicine is still too Empirical ....We are still relying on observations rather than on rational arguments to understand the insensible operations of the sensible parts ... And often we find it difficult to decide on the process of passing from a healthy to an unhealthy state, or from illness to health; in other words, we hesitate over the causes of and the treatments for diseases.[32]

We need therefore to understand the conditions under which Leibniz can envisage the legitimate use of experimentation in medicine. What is interesting here is the realization that, for Leibniz, it is precisely the recourse to experience when constituting this field of learning that makes it difficult to decide between health and illness, to the extent that if medicine as based solely on rational arguments we would be able to identify the causes of diseases and their cures with certainty.

Empirical Medicine: A Provisional Body of Knowledge?

It would appear, therefore, that considering empirical medicine as legitimate is justified provided that medical observations are taken as a

---

[32] Sarah Carvallo, *Stahl-Leibniz, Controverse sur le vivant, l'organisme et le mixte* (Paris, 2004), 113.

provisional substitute for intangible knowledge of the causes. This lack of knowledge is the result of the fact that medicine is still in the early stages of development—Leibniz in fact writes that "this special physics is barely in the cradle."[33] He is obviously at pains here to distance himself from the positions of the ancient "Empirical Medicine," which opposed "dogmatic" medicine by rejecting any attempt to determine the hidden causes of disease, limiting itself to identifying symptoms. In a text dated 1702, Leibniz very explicitly makes this distinction but, interestingly, mentions a third option:

> In medicine, there are the sect of the Empiricists and those of Method and of Reason. The first allowed no seeking of causes or reasons, being satisfied solely with facts or experiments, as if saying: this was either profitable or harmful, and thus can still be either profitable or harmful in a similar case. Those who simply followed Method had no concern for observations or experiments, they believed that they had reduced everything to the causes or reasons. But the physicians following Reason attempted to perfect the experiment by also searching for the causes.[34]

This third option indicates, in my view, the status that Leibniz explicitly attributes to medical experiments: "perfect the experiment by also searching for the causes."[35] It is in this sense that I believe we can speak of a 'provisional empiricism'. I use this expression to refer to what Leibniz, in a fragment of text from 1678-1680 entitled *De notionibus empiricis*, describes as provisional definitions which alone can be adequate to empirical notions.[36]

---

[33] G.W. Leibniz, *Animadversiones*, Responsiones, ad §11, ed. Dutens, *Opera omnia* (Geneva, 1767), II-2,148: "Sed haec minus mirari debemus, quia Physica specialis omnis fere hactenus in cunis jacet."

[34] Comments by Leibniz on an extract from the article "Rorarius" in the text of 1702 already mentioned (*GP* IV, 525-26).

[35] As in the short text already cited, *Veritates physicae*, Leibniz, by referring to mixed truths, describes the practice of reasonable physicians: "VERITATES MIXTAE sunt quae partim ex sensualibus partim ex intellectualibus concluduntur" (*A* VI, 4, 1984).

[36] *Nouveaux Essais* (*A*, VI, 6, 299-300) and "De Notionibus empiricis" (*A*, VI, 4, 16): "In *Notionibus Empiricis*, ut auri, et aliorum in quibus de possibilitate non constat nisi a posteriori; non habentur definitiones nisi provisionales." Cf. on this subject Christian Leduc's excellent analysis in the last part of chapter 5 of *Substance, individu et connaissance chez Leribniz* (Montreal, 2009).

This is what gives Leibniz' position its force: the value of experiments in medicine can be recognized provided they are regarded as a simple stage in the development of a field of knowledge which will eventually be able to positively identify the causes of diseases. The question is, what kind of knowledge is yielded by this provisional skill?

While at one level, medical experiments are accepted as making a provisional contribution of skills that are useful to human health, which potentially, but not yet actually, amounts to empiricism, Leibniz appears to go a little further, and this is where the examination becomes delicate.

Leibniz here seems to be taking a middle ground between two positions. On the one hand, there is the recourse to experimentation—in a sense, conceded—until it can be replaced by true knowledge which will be based on the identification of the causes of diseases. On the other, a model of truth conceived as the interface between observation and reasoning. On this latter point, I refer to §19, book IV, ch.7 of the *Nouveaux Essais*. After pointing out that M. Barner had envisioned a method of explaining the art of healing that, rather than considering diseases one after another according to the order of the parts of the human body, "could start from universal precepts of practice common to several diseases or symptoms," Leibniz adds:

> I believe that he is right to advise this method, especially concerning those precepts where *medicine is ratiocinative*; but the more *empirical* medicine is, the less easy and the less safe it is to form universal propositions. [...] Thus, notwithstanding the universal precepts, it is wise to seek among the types of diseases, cures and remedies that satisfy multiple indications and causes taken together, and particularly to use those that have proved themselves through experiment. In medicine, the principles of experience, that is to say, the observations, cannot be too numerous, so as to allow our reason more opportunity to decipher what nature only half reveals to us.[37]

In this passage, Leibniz points out the need to draw from both experience and abstract reasoning in constituting remedies. Note the elegant expression "principles of experience" used to describe observations. Once again, he urges their multiplication, this time explaining why: "to allow our

---

[37] Leibniz, *Nouveaux Essais sur l'entendement humain*, book IV, ch. 7, § 19, 336, ed. Jacques Brunschwig (Paris, 1990).

reason more opportunity to decipher what nature only half reveals to us."[38] Naturally, his first concern here is to justify experimentation as the means to a possible deciphering of nature. There is a theme at work here similar to that used by Leibniz to describe chemical operations. Elsewhere, he refers to the production or discovery of new bodies by the chemists as a kind of *foretaste*, insofar as it revealed the imperceptible, which only becomes visible through either the use of the microscope or our later discovery of the causes.

This interpretation is consistent with Duchesneau's findings in *Physiologie des Lumières: empirisme, modèles et theories*:

> Leibniz adds that, since the inner workings of the organic processes are hidden to our view beyond a certain level of observation, the analogy linking the processes of phenomena according to the suggestions of experience can give us a foretaste of the mechanical sufficient reason behind the processes.[39]

While this concept of acting on nature in order to know it emerges fully here, what Leibniz means when he writes that "nature only half reveals certain things to us" remains to be clarified. In my view, this phrase clearly draws an outline or provides a frame, even, for this provisional empiricism, both furnishing a justification for the recourse to experimentation and setting the limits for such recourse: it becomes an instrument to be employed in the work of reason, which will use it to arrive at the causes of diseases. §11 in the same chapter develops this point while drawing a parallel between theology and medicine:

> It is like saying: medicine is founded on experience, therefore reason plays no part in it. Christian theology, which is the true medicine of the soul, is founded on revelation which evokes experience, but in order for it to become complete it needs to be linked to natural theology derived from the axioms of eternal reason.[40]

While Leibniz recognizes the need to rely on experiment in medicine, he nonetheless considers that, in order for medicine to be complete as a body of knowledge, it has to use reason. This is, at least, how I interpret

---

38) *Ibid.*
39) Duchesneau, *Physiologie des Lumières*, 90.
40) Leibniz, *Nouveaux Essais*, 327.

the interplay between analysis and synthesis Leibniz uses in the text of 1680-2 *De scribendis novis Medicinae Elementis*, which was first translated into French by Duchesneau in an appendix to *Leibniz, le vivant et l'organisme*.[41]

Practical Medicine: A Field of Learning Situated between Analysis and Synthesis

After pointing out, first, that writing in medicine amounts to no more than prescribing for a machine the method that will preserve its health, and second, that if we imagine the workings of this machine rather than drawing it out from experience then we have little hope of advancing medicine, Leibniz illustrates twice in this short text how analysis and synthesis are complementary in the cognitive method of medicine.[42] What does he mean here by these terms?

Leibniz describes the method as analytical insofar as it seeks the means or the organs of a given function and their ways of operating, thus arriving at an understanding of the body through its parts. Here, we may be approaching the project for a real alphabet, set up for the analysis of the use of microscopic observation in medicine. Anatomical analysis is the way to constitute such a 'real alphabet'. For the argument to be complete, however, we need to return to synthesis; that is, to describing all the parts co-ordinated within a body and the full system of the animal, especially if we have learned through analysis the organs relevant to each function.

Thus, the fragmentation of the body described by Mandressi is not yet accepted by Leibniz within this scheme, which is attempting to maintain at the same time both the *resolutio ad minutum* and the integrity of the body. This passage ends by distinguishing between three functions of the bodily parts: "all the parts of our body can be distinguished as being what contains, what is contained and what is an agent of impetus, that is in veins, humours and spirits, and thus our body is a hydraulico-pneumatico-pyrobolic machine."[43]

---

[41] Duchesneau, *Leibniz, le vivant et l'organisme*, 312-17.

[42] Cf. Duchesneau, *Leibniz, le vivant et l'organisme*, 312.

[43] On preserving the health of a machine, see *ibid.*, 314.

This play between analysis and synthesis is used again in the last lines of the text to distinguish between two methods of treating illnesses. One method is analytic and deals with symptoms, the other synthetic and deals with causes. This is the starting point. However, "what should be taught is true analysis, that is, on the one hand the art of studying the signs, and on the other, the art of inferring the disease from these signs. Synthesis should be taught after a model of analysis has been presented, that is, a model of a general method of treatment whih is to pathological synthesis what algebra is to the elements of geometry."[44]

This medical semiology is of course rather striking. Clearly, signs or symptoms are to be identified and used as a means of discovering the causes of illnesses, the diseases themselves. Equally striking, however, is the fact that Leibniz is in fact setting out the possibility of a real link between empirical medicine and rational medicine. This possibility, it would seem, is made effective by the idea that analysis is capable of identifying causes. In so doing, Leibniz is blurring the traditional distinction between the empirical analytic method and the rational synthetic method because he is proposing an analytical method that makes it possible to trace the causes of symptoms provisionally; that is to say, subject to other symptoms altering the identification of the causes. The analogy between algebra, analysis and synthesis on the one hand, and the elements of geometry on the other, has been used, in my opinion, to reveal the status of this analysis: an alphabet that can enable us to identify the real, though invisible, constituents of the human body.

Experimentation: A Perceptive Foretaste or the Condition for the Advancement of Knowledge?

Referring to the *Directiones ad rem medicam pertinentes* and working from the text I have just explored, which defines analysis "as the art of studying the signs and inferring the disease from these signs," I intend to show that this action on the body, this penetration of the body (via the analysis of anaesthesia, the autopsy or, in a somewhat different perspective, digestion, and so on), promises an intelligibility that is both provisional and unequalled. To act on the body in order to understand it seems

---

[44] *Ibid.*, 317.

to constitute, to Leibniz' eyes, the epistemological challenge of the practice of medical experimentation. Provided it is regarded as a provisional substitute for knowledge, medical experimentation offers a true *perceptive foretaste,* hinting at the certainty of the knowledge to come. The experiments on the body that Leibniz describes in this text from 1671 are presented as ways of rendering visible what we do not understand. In the following section I will discuss two examples of this: one is the description of the merits of the autopsy and the other speaks highly of animal experimentation.

Visibility and Intelligibility

Before commenting on this text, I would like to point out that it centres on the description of practices useful in learning about the human body. Basically, it consists of descriptions of ways of measuring perspiration or the size of humans, of weighing, distilling, clarifying urine and blood; it includes paragraphs on the need to understand how quickly a liquid reaches the stomach after consumption as a function of its degree of acidity, diets that lead to longer life. There are also, however, experiments describing the effect in terms of life expectancy of a sedentary way of life, or of giving a man first only water, then water and bread, and so on, or of transfusion experiments: he suggests injecting a variety of liquids into the blood and gives the example of a weak horse who gained weight after receiving the blood of a young ewe.

Let us provide two examples here.[45] The first is a detailed description of the questions that should be addressed to the body when practising an autopsy. For example, try to understand what it is that is eating away the flesh while leaving all the ducts intact. Here, the challenge is explicit: through the extreme precision of the examination, to obtain a "living anatomy"; that is, to open up dead bodies and, through the questions that are answered by this opening up, to understand the living body as a whole.

---

[45] G.W. Leibniz, "Directions pertaining to the Institution of Medicine (1671)," *Leibnizhandschriften* (LH) III, 1, 3, folio 1-9, manuscript translated by Justin Smith in *Divine Machines,* 275-287.

The second example concerns animal experimentation, which is "analogous with the human body." Leibniz' thesis here is the importance of comparative anatomy and of experimentation on animals: their bodies can be opened up whenever and however we wish; medicines can also be tested on animals, allowing useful conclusions to be drawn, by analogy, for human beings.

In these two examples, experimentation appears to me to be clearly that act whereby opening up bodies, dead bodies or animal bodies, is made explicitly the means of understanding the living body as a whole. This penetration of bodies, being unique as a means of learning, is a perceptive foretaste insofar as it creates the conditions of legibility of what we are trying to find out and cannot, for the moment, find out otherwise. Of course, in an existential sense, there is a kind of tragic irony in conceiving of death as a way of obtaining a foretaste of our future knowledge of life, in searching the dead body for the encrypted key to the living body. Despite all this, the idea of a heuristic resolution is being formulated here. Whether this *resolutio* is retrospective or comparative (regarding animal testing), it is part of the same conviction: that bodily dissection can provide a foretaste of knowledge of the body. The crucial question is whether it is in this sense alone that such an empirical body of learning is provisional.

The Status of the Perceptive Foretaste in the Conception of Knowledge

The question here is this: how should this perceptive foretaste, or to put it differently, this 'provisional empiricism', be understood? We have clearly established an initial understanding of provisional empiricism as being founded on the possibility of constituting a real alphabet:

First, something resembling a provisional empiricism has been identified through examining: (i) the explicit and partially realized project for collecting observations; (ii) the use of the microscope as an instrument of analysis which simultaneously enhances visibility and comprehension; (iii) the description of experiments on bodies to make them comprehensible; and (iv) the classification of these experiments and observations under the category of induction. Second, this empiricism has been shown to be provisional to the extent that Leibniz explicitly describes it as a way of understanding something prior to achieving a rational grasp of it, while waiting to grasp it rationally, which is what I have called a 'perceptive foretaste'. Third, this 'perceptive foretaste' also comes into play in defining the status of chemistry: it provides an interesting and, to some extent, unprecedented image of intelligibility in Leibnizian natural philosophy.

This alphabet, or systematic overview, confers a form of universality on sensible truths and legitimacy on the aspiration to identify the causes through analysis. We can therefore identify a provisional empiricism specific to a mixed system of knowledge which links experience and reason, like the 'reasonable physicians'.

There is also, however, a second meaning of provisional empiricism which, in line with the highly evocative suggestions by Leduc attributes to this knowledge founded on experience the capacity to evolve through contact with new experiences that might alter our knowledge. In this respect, the question is whether this other face of cognitive practice, explicitly outlined by Leibniz, does not in fact propose a more flexible version of empiricism than those contemporary with it.[46]

Ultimately, the challenge is to understand the connection between these two meanings of 'provisional empiricism': between knowledge that is provisional because it is based on experience that is necessarily less certain than reasoning, and knowledge that is provisional because further experience is likely to perfect it. In other words, one view of experiments as lacking in rationality, and the other which sees experimentation as the condition for the advancement of knowledge. I would suggest that what is present here is more than a tension, and can be understood from the perspective adopted by Leibniz: in his epistemological set-up, provisional empiricism necessarily takes its place as one stage in the rational ordering of the world, but from the 'practical' perspective that we often see Leibniz adopting, it can be considered a condition for the advancement of knowledge.

---

[46] Leduc, *Substance, individu et connaissance chez Leibniz*, ch. 5.

Whytt and the Idea of Power:
Physiological Evidence as a Challenge to the Eighteenth-Century Criticism of the Notion of Power

Claire Etchegaray

University of Paris X (Paris-Nanterre-La Defense) *

Abstract

In *An Essay on the Vital and Involuntary Motions of Animals*, Robert Whytt maintained that the muscular motions that perform the natural functions of the organism are caused by an immaterial power. Here we consider to what extent the philosophical criticism of power urged by Locke and Hume may jeopardize his thesis, how his response mobilizes the resources of the Scottish experimental theism and whether he makes an original use of such resources. First, we examine various pieces of experimental evidence from which Whytt infers the need to evoke this power, before showing how they prompt him to stand by the immaterial power in the face of the empiricist criticisms. Following this, we explore the link Whytt makes between power and agency, in particular comparing his thought with Locke's. Lastly, we examine his work in the light of Hume's criticism regarding the question of whether a power may be felt.

Keywords

active principles, agency, animism, William Cullen, experimental method, feeling, Albrecht von Haller, David Hume, Francis Hutcheson, John Locke, materialism, nerves, power, Thomas Reid, Scottish Enlightenment, soul, sympathy, Robert Whytt

Whytt's Medical Project in the *Essay*

In 1744, dissatisfied with the widespread theories of cardiac motion and respiration, Robert Whytt began to write the *Essay on the Vital and other Involuntary Motions of Animals*.[1] In the volume that he eventually pub-

---

* Institut de Recherches Philosophiques (IREPH), University of Paris X (Paris-Nanterre-La Defense), 200 avenue de la République, 92001 Nanterre, France (claire.etchegaray@u-paris10.fr).

lished in 1751, he used the hypothesis of the action of an immaterial power present in the nerves to explain the motions by which bodily functions are performed.[2] He opposed the materialism and mechanism that, according to him, Albrecht von Haller's conception of the fibre might entail. Julien Offray de la Mettrie had translated Haller's annotation to Herman Boerhaave's *Institutiones medicae* into French in 1743 and dedicated *L'homme machine* to the physician of Göttingen in 1748. In the *Essay*, Whytt alleges that the opinion that there is an inherent property of contraction in the muscular fibre paves the way for an unknown material and mechanistic cause of animal motion. He takes this opinion, defended by Haller, to be a "refuge of ignorance." But couldn't this accusation have been applied to Whytt himself: couldn't the appeal to an immaterial power have been taken as a "refuge of ignorance" too? Intending to shed light on the anthropological implications of Whytt's position, in addition to his contribution to the history of neurophysiology, scholars' interest has focused on three main areas: his metaphysical presuppositions, the sociological background to the concept of *sensibility* and *sympathy* and the coherence of his Newtonian approach.[3]

---

[1] Robert Whytt, *An Essay on the Vital and Involuntary Motions of Animals* (Edinburgh, 1751, second ed. with corrections and additions, Edinburgh, 1763).

[2] Roger Kenneth French, *Robert Whytt. The Soul and Medicine* (London, 1969).

[3] On the history of neurophysiology, see Georges Canguilhem, *La formation du concept de réflexe aux XVIIe et XVIIIe siècles* (Paris, 1955), 101-106; Eugenio Frixione, "Irritable Glue: The Haller-Whytt Controversy on the Mechanism of Muscle Contraction," in Harry Whitaker, Christopher U.M. Smith and Stanley Finger, eds, *Brain, Mind and Medicine* (Marquette, Birmingham, St. Louis, 2007), 115-24; and Max Neuburger, *The Historical Development of Experimental Brain and Spinal Cord Physiology Before Flourens* (Baltimore and London, 1981). On the metaphysical theses, see John P. Wright, "Metaphysics and Physiology: Mind, Body and the Animal Economy in the Eighteenth Century Scotland," in M. A. Stewart, ed., *Studies in the Philosophy of the Scottish Enlightenment* (Oxford, 1990; reprinted 2000), 251-301; and John P. Wright, "Substance versus Function Dualism in Eighteenth Century Medicine," in John P. Wright and Paul Potter, eds., *Psyche and Soma. Physicians and Metaphysicians on the Mind-Body Problem from Antiquity to Enlightenment* (Oxford, 2000; reprinted 2007), 253-54. On the sociological background, see Christopher Lawrence, "The Nervous System and Society in the Scottish Enlightenment," in Barry Barnes and Steven Shapin, eds., *Natural Order. Historical Studies in Scientific Culture* (Beverly Hills, 1979), 19-40. On the Newtonian approach, see François Duchesneau, *La physiologie des Lumières. Empirisme, modèles et théories* (The Hague, Boston and London, 1982), 171-215.

Our aim in this article is to examine Whytt's notion of power, for Lockean and Humean criticisms suggest its irrelevance. Yet as John P. Wright points out, the experimental method was currently being promoted in Scotland by the "Rankenian Club." Whytt's own teacher, George Young, was a member of this club, founded around 1716, which was circulating an experimental theism and discussing George Berkeley's, Samuel Clarke's and Isaac Newton's thoughts. The interesting questions are, therefore, to what extent Whytt may have been responding to the philosophical objections urged by Locke and Hume, in what way the resources of the Scottish experimental theism are expedient in his physiological approach and whether he makes an original use of such resources. We shall firstly recall Whytt's original theses before examining the metaphysical reasons for his position from the Lockean and Humean points of view.

The First Experimental Evidence for an Immaterial Power in the *Essay*

The experimental method used by Whytt is qualified in the advertisement by implicit reference to the Newtonian rules of philosophizing.[4] Rejecting hypotheses entails assuming plain facts, that is to say facts that are causes, proved to be existent and not more complicated than their effects. Their features are uniformity and simplicity.[5] Thus, because some facts are regularly linked to others, we are justified in inferring causes. Simplicity has to be understood in methodological, ontological and psychological ways. Indeed, identifying the cause does not depend on knowledge of its essence; the cause merely resides in the power to produce particular phenomena, and that is all we can say about it. Being unique and sufficient to produce its effect, the cause provides the psychological satisfaction of an "easy solution." Yet causality is not so easy

---

[4] Isaac Newton, *The* Principia: *the Mathematical Principles of Natural Philosophy*, ed. I. Bernard Cohen (Berkeley CA, 1999), Book III.

[5] This is why Whytt rejects any monstrous evidence: "No reasoning drawn from a few monstrous cases, can be sufficient to overthrow a doctrine founded upon the plainest *phaenomena* observed in perfect animals, and confirmed by almost numberless experiments made upon them" (Whytt, *Essay*, section 1, 8).

to discern: the complexity of phenomena may conceal it from the naïve observer.

The first experimental support for an immaterial power stems from the first of the plain facts given at the beginning of the *Essay*:

> A certain power or influence proceeding originally from the brain and spinal marrow, lodged afterwards in the nerves, and by their means conveyed into the muscles, is either the immediate cause of their contraction, or at least necessary to it.[6]

The power is not yet described as immaterial in the first section. Although in the first half of the book Whytt increasingly confirms the role of a nervous power that is not purely mechanical, he makes this immateriality clear only in accounting for the sympathetic phenomena of respiratory motions (in the middle of the book). The requisite simplicity justifies the assumption of a single and general explanatory power. In the introduction, Whytt warns against any attempt "to explain the vital motions of almost every different organ by a different theory."[7] Thus, he asserts a single "energy" operating throughout the chain of causes and effects involved in the contraction of the muscle, for he subscribes to the thesis that causality in bodies needs active powers of some sort. In this respect, he agrees with other Scottish physicians including, as pointed out in Whytt's notebook, his teacher George Young. Young had already expressed dissatisfaction with the Boerhaavean hypothesis and the "free Influx" explanation of the muscular motions, stating that the cause of the dilatation of the muscle might not be exclusively mechanical. Young also regarded the application of special laws in bodies as being "in virtue of their being animated by an immaterial spirit."[8] Whytt himself thinks that he is justified in appealing to a non-mechanical and non-material cause that exerts its power throughout the bodily parts.

The notion of influence precludes any deterministic reading of this assumption. As attested by its astrological connotation, it refers to a cau-

---

[6] Whytt, *Essay*, 5.

[7] Whytt, *Essay*, 4-5.

[8] Wright, "Metaphysics and Physiology," 277-280. Whytt's notebook was based on his studies with George Young. The two notes quoted by Wright are entitled "Of muscular motion" (431 ff.) and "Of sensation" (467 ff.), in George Young, *Lectures on Medicine. Taken by Robert Whytt. Edinburgh, 1730-31 40*, Royal College of Physician of Edinburgh, MS. M9.19.

sality that is different from its effect *by nature*. The contraction is not merely an effect of the nervous power caused by cerebral power, since in some monstrous instances contractions and sensations remain despite the deficiency of the brain. The vicariousness suggests that, throughout the causal chain, one and the same power exerts its influence, to which no material origin can be assigned. Even the expressions "animal spirits" and "vital spirits," that Young had already criticized,[9] are only names by which this power is denoted, not notions explanatory of it.

The second piece of experimental evidence in support of such a power is found in the explanation of the circulation of the blood. From Stephen Hales' experiments on the *momentum* of the blood, Whytt infers that the Boerhaavean principles are not sufficient to explain the alternating contraction of the heart and the force by which the blood is diffused in all the veins and arteries.[10] According to Boerhaave, at the end of the systole, when the auricles and arteries are distended by blood, the nerves that are between them should be compressed so that the animal spirits are trapped in nerves; this, Whytt argues, would mean that the heart would be rendered "paralytic."[11] Then its cavities are relaxed, the blood flows out and the nervous fluids circulate again. Whytt objects that *since nerves are hollow pipes*, either the spirits cause contraction by being injected into the fibres of muscles and then, once they are no longer trapped, being pushed into the fibres of the heart, which results in its contraction rather than *diastole*; or, the inflow of the spirits does not cause any contraction of the heart,[12] which leaves the phenomena unexplained. Given the hydraulic hypotheses, no mechanical explanation can account for the alternating cardiac motion. Referring to Glisson,[13] Whytt argues that "the contraction of the heart is not solely owing to its fibres being distracted by the moment of the blood, but partly to the irritation communicated to its internal surface by the particles of that fluid."[14] But, again, the irritation does not cause contraction by the weight and the

---

[9] Wright, "Metaphysics and Physiology," 277-80.

[10] Roger Kenneth French, "Sauvages, Whytt and the motion of the heart: aspect of eighteenth-century animism," *Clio Medica*, 7 (1972), 34-54.

[11] Whytt, *Essay*, 49.

[12] *Ibid.*, section 3.

[13] Francis Glisson, *Tractatus de ventriculo et intestinis* (London, 1677), ch. 7.

[14] Whytt, *Essay*, 53.

influx of blood. Whytt conceives of *stimulation* as an original fact; that is, in the context of the Scottish Enlightenment, a fact which cannot be explained other than by appeal to "the constitution of our nature." He thinks that stimulation is an energy produced after affection by virtue of our constitution, and that affection entails sensibility by virtue of the very same constitution. This very point will give rise to the dispute with Haller in the future *Physiological Essays* (published in 1755): Whytt thinks that no irritation can be stimulation without entailing sensibility, whereas Haller holds that irritation and sensibility are two distinct powers, linked respectively to muscular fibre and to nervous fibre.[15] Yet they agree that no inquiry into the structure or the "fabrick" of the fibre can account for an original phenomenon of this nature. In these *Physiological essays*, Whytt's views rest on various experiments: small pox and acrid food increase the motion of the blood, applying an acrid substance to the heart renews its contraction, etc. The role of the nerves is induced from a huge set of experimental facts too. The "constitution and peculiar sensibility" of them is the main cause, but cannot be explained by the material frame and mechanical function of the animal spirits. The notion of "original affection" was familiar to the Rankenian members and their followers, due to their interest in Hutcheson's moral philosophy. The latter claimed, in the preface of *An Inquiry into the Original of Our Ideas of Beauty and Virtue* (published in 1725), that:

> The presence of some objects necessarily pleases us, and the presence of others as necessarily displeases us. [...] By the very frame of our nature, the one is made the occasion of delight, and the other of dissatisfaction.[16]

In Hutcheson's view, the "frame of nature" does not mean the material constitution of our body. The expression refers to the essence of what we are, as created beings. It is an ontological notion connected to the thesis of the chain of beings or *naturae scala*. Given our metaphysically unknown nature, the presence of an object can be either delightful or disagreeable. Now Whytt uses the assumption of sensibility as a fact of nature in a medical context in order to subvert mechanical and material

---

[15] Robert Whytt, *Physiological Essays* (Edinburgh, [1755] 1761).
[16] Francis Hutcheson, *An Inquiry into the Original of the Ideas of Beauty and Virtue in Two Treatises* (Indianapolis, 2004), preface, 8.

theories. This emerges particularly strongly in the explanation of respiration. The problem faced by the physiologist in explaining respiration is to understand "by what power or mechanism inspiration and expiration alternately succeed each other, or why the intercostal muscles and diaphragm are contracted and relaxed by turns, so long as life remains."[17] Boerhaave's theory explained the relaxation of muscles in expiration mechanically. But Whytt is intrigued by the passage from expiration to inspiration. His hypothesis is once again that the motions of the thorax proceed from a stimulus or an uneasy sensation in the lungs that "accompanies the difficult passage of the blood thro' the pulmonary vessels." Yet the story doesn't end there, because we still need to explain how this sensation in the lungs can affect different, independent parts of the thorax: the intercostal muscles, the diaphragm and even the abdominal organs. They are all set in motion together. At first, a mere nervous connection (called sympathy) between each of these independent organs is conjectured; but no such material connection is observed, even in the brain. So Whytt is led to rethink the medical notion of sympathy as a fact of an original nature. In *An Essay on the Nature and Conduct of the Passions and Affections with Illustrations on the Moral Sense* (published in 1728), Hutcheson had already asserted that sympathy is an effect of the constitution of our nature.[18] Whytt, however, connects sympathy with an active power, that is, the power of an agency that cannot be material:

> The sympathy, therefore, or consent observed between the nerves of various parts of the body, is not to be explained mechanically, but ought to be ascribed to the energy of that sentient being, which in a peculiar manner displays its powers in the brain, and, by means of the nerves, moves, actuates, and enlivens the whole machine.[19]

This recourse to the "energy of a sentient being" is confirmed by various experiments and is explicit in the rest of the book. After a section on the beginning of respiration in the foetus, the last sections examine the role of this energy in stimulation, and more generally the role of the spirit in involuntary motions. In this context, Whytt regards the account of stim-

---

[17] Whytt, *Essay*, section 8, 200.
[18] Hutcheson, *An Essay on the Nature*, I.i.3.
[19] Whytt, *Essay*, section 8, 204.

ulus by a "latent power" in the fibre as a "refuge of ignorance." The following constitutes the first attack against Haller, whose annotation of Boerhaave is quoted in footnote:

> But this opinion seems to be no more than a refuge of ignorance, which nothing, but the despair of any success in their inquiries into this matter, can have driven into. For if they [Haller and other defenders of any "latent power"] here mean some unknown active powers resulting from the peculiar constitution or mechanical structure of a muscular fibre, it may be sufficient reason with us for denying there are any such latent causes, that the assertors of them have hitherto been as unable to vindicate their existence by *phaenomena* which cannot be explained without them, as to specify their true nature; besides that it must appear greatly unphilosophical to attribute active powers to that, which however modified or arranged is yet no more than a system of mere matter ; powers I say, which are not only confessedly superior to the utmost effort of mechanism, but seemingly contrary to all the known properties of matter.[20]

Now, it appears that Whytt's accusation stems from his conception of the active powers. Attributing to a material object (the fibre) such an "active," "hidden" power endows matter with power that is foreign to any quality that can be observed in it. In the end, the two decisive features of Whytt's conception of power seem to be its connection to *agency* and its property of being *felt*:

> Some may, perhaps, be of opinion, that the all-wise Author of nature hath endued the muscular fibres of animals with certain active powers, far superior to those of common matter, and that to these the motions of irritated muscles are owing. And indeed we cannot but readily acknowledge, that he has animated all the muscles and fibres of animals, with an active sentient principle united to their bodies, and that, to the energy of this principles, are owing, the contractions of stimulated muscles. But if it be imagined that he has given to animal fibres a power of sensation, and of generating motion, without superadding or uniting to them an active principle, as the subject and cause of these, we presume to say, that a supposition of this kind ought by no means be admitted; since, to affirm that matter can, of itself, by any modification of its parts, be rendered capable of sensation, or of generating motion, is not less absurd, than to ascribe to it a power of thinking.[21]

---

[20] *Ibid.*, 266-67.
[21] *Ibid.*, 268.

As these features might be contradicted by the previous analyses of the idea of "power" in the philosophical studies of the understanding led by Locke and Hume, we shall turn to them.[22] Actually, Whytt does not explicitly discuss Lockean and Humean views. His hypotheses could, however, be seen either as an indulgent return to the occult quality, or as a striking instance of how the physician refined notions previously analysed by the philosophy of the mind. Before dealing with this point it should be noted that, rather than getting involved in metaphysical debate, Whytt considers possible physiological objections. Couldn't the organic functions be said to be insensible, at least at certain regular and vital times; e.g., in sleep? He sets out his answer in sections XII and XIII. This was an important issue for Whytt, as attested by his personal papers.[23] Section XIII was published for the second time in 1754 in a separate article.[24] Since "[t]he heart can only be affected by stimuli, in so far as it is a sentient organ—i.e., endued with feeling"—how can it be possible for blood circulation and respiration to go on in sleep? He answers that "[i]n ordinary sleep, the sensibility of the heart and lungs suffer so small a diminution, that their motions will be very little more affected by it, than they would be from the horizontal position and rest of the body, and composure of mind attending it"; whereas in morbid sleep or

---

[22] In the following, I do not discuss Locke's hypothesis of thinking matter. As is well known, he introduces this notion in a text, which Whytt might implicitly echo, as follows: "It being, in respect of our notions, not much more remote from our comprehension to conceive, that God can, if he pleases, superadd to matter a faculty of thinking, than that he should superadd to it another substance, with a faculty of thinking; since we know not wherein thinking consists, nor to what sort of substances the Almighty has been pleased to give that power, which cannot be in any created being, but merely by the good pleasure and Bounty of the creator" (John Locke, *Essay concerning Human Understanding*, ed. P.H. Nidditch (Oxford, 1975), IV.iii.6).

[23] In a personal manuscript, Whytt flattered himself with having reduced the "question concerning the seat of soul" "to physical problem" experimentally solved. But he confessed: "There are two considerable points however which I have not yet treated of, without which the account which I gave of the brain and nerves must be imperfect; I mean the manner in which muscular motion is performed by the nerves & and the nature of sleep." (*Manuscripts*, Wellcome Institute of the History of Medicine).

[24] "Of the difference between Respiration and the motion of the Heart, in sleeping and waking persons," in *Essays and Observations, Physical and Literary* (Edinburgh, 1754), 492-503.

in sleep artificially caused by opium, the lesser degree of sensibility leads to a slowness of the pulse. It seems that the sensibility *of an organ* ("sensibility of the heart," "sensibility of the lungs") is conditioned by the general exercise of the sentient principle. But Whytt does not detail how the degree of local sensibility is related to the degree of exertion of the sentient power in the whole body, nor does he explain how different scales of intensity and pleasure of sensibility are interrelated or related to health—probably because the general sympathy as well as the particular feeling remain facts of nature in his view.

From a Lockean Point of View

Why is the "opinion, that the all-wise Author of nature hath endued the muscular fibres of animals with certain active powers" not sufficiently well-defined? The notion of "active power" left room for various ways of theorizing physical powers because it had a threefold connotation: Neoplatonic plastic nature, a chemical interpretation, traceable to Van Helmont, and dissatisfaction with the mere passive role of matter in mechanical post-Cartesian accounts. The English tradition assumed active principles either by asserting them as *inherent* to matter or by arguing that they act *on* the matter.[25] Whytt's position clearly precludes the first option: indeed, according to him, the recent experimental observations of the energy at work in circulation and respiration are sufficient grounds for believing that an active power is required, because matter has exclusively passive powers.[26] The second option is more problematic. John Wright has recalled that the origin of Whytt's notion of an immaterial active cause may be found in Newton's *Opticks* and in the correspondence between Samuel Clarke and Leibniz. Newton thinks that there is a "necessity of conserving and recruiting [the variety of Motion in the World] by active Principles, such as are the Cause of Gravity [...] and the cause of fermentation by which the heart and blood of animals are kept

---

[25] John Henry, "Occult Qualities and the Experimental Philosophy: Active Principles in Pre-Newtonian Matter Theory," *History of Science*, 24 (1986), 335-81.

[26] At least Whytt cannot be accused of supposing a real accident in matter. See René Descartes, Letter to Elisabeth dated the 21st of May, 1643, in *Oeuvres philosophiques III* (Paris, 1989), 21.

in perpetual motion and heat."[27] Clarke argues that the creator must constantly intervene in nature and that motion cannot be perpetual and increasing unless it is by "a principle of life and activity."[28] Nonetheless, as long as this intervention is conceived as that of a transcendant almighty, the model of the body can remain a machine. However, if the active principle is inherent to the life of the body, the object of medicine ceases to be a mere machine and becomes the subject of the power. For Whytt, the living body is not simply an automatic machine activated by an external active power. Actually, he came to this conclusion after years of study: in his early lectures he defended the model of a machine externally animated.[29] Later, however, in a passage of the *Essay* quoted above, he can be seen to hold the human body to be an *enlivened* machine.

Now comes the objection. Whytt might be suspected of introducing a "substantial form" within the living body by defending the existence of an immaterial being that is the *agent* of involuntary motions. Locke had already condemned this kind of error.[30] The experimental method that he advocated in medical matters means renouncing enquiry into hidden causes, those Galenic faculties or virtues, which were considered in metaphysics as real accidents or substantial forms. It is well known that Locke shared with Thomas Sydenham the view that the physician should describe sensible patterns of diseases, uniformly produced by nature,

---

[27] Newton, *Opticks*, 398-99. See. James E. McGuire, *Tradition and Innovation: Newton's Metaphysics of Nature*, ch. 5 (Dordrecht, 1995), ch. 5; and Andrew Janiak, *Newton as Philosopher* (Cambridge 2003), chs. 3 and 4.

[28] Henry G. Alexander, ed., *The Leibniz-Clarke Correspondence* (Manchester, 1956), 112.

[29] "As the infinite wisdom and power of the deity are manifestly apparent in all his works, (the heavens declaring his glory and firmanent shewing forth his handy work), so no where are they more conspicuous, no where more to be admired, than in the composure of the humane machine for what an infinity of vessels of various sizes & different natures do we have behold!," Whytt, *Manuscripts*, Wellcome Institute of the History of Medicine, MS 6861/46-47, *Insensible perspiration*. This might be a variant of the argument labelled "Galen's muscles" by Isabel Rivers ("'Galen's Muscles': Wilkins, Hume and the Educational Use of the Argument from Design," *The Historical Journal*, 36 (1993), 577-97.).

[30] See also Robert Boyle, *The Origin of Forms and Qualities*, in Thomas Birch, ed. *The Works* (Hildesheim, 1966), Cf. Bruno Gnassounou and Max Kistler, *Dispositions and Causal Powers* (Aldershot, 2007), 7-16.

without imagining any substantial causality.[31] Furthermore, explicit mention of the medical irrelevance of the concept of "faculty" can be found in the chapter "Of Power" in the *Essay concerning Human Understanding* (§ 20). According to Locke, an active power is a power of *changing* or of *interrupting* and, as such, of *beginning*. It belongs to an *agent*. But we must carefully prevent any multiplication of hidden causes by avoiding supposing different agents for each capacity. Locke thinks that the sole "clear idea" of beginning an action, either of motion or thought, is that of the will or of the power of perception. Thus, will and understanding are the only powers that an agent can experience by reflection. Whether this agent is the man or the mind is not the point. Locke's conviction is that there can only be one agent: the one who feels the power. A notable consequence stems from this: the term "faculty" cannot denote any *agent* in the mind or the body. It only denotes a power. Echoing this paragraph of Locke's *Essay* in the *Cyclopedia* first published in 1728, Chambers denounces "this practice of attributing effect to their respective virtue or *faculties*," such as accounting for the act of digestion by supposing a "digestive faculty in the stomach," or for motion by imagining "a *motive faculty* in the nerves": "A FACULTY of *an animal body*, is defined to be the principle whereby the body performs its functions."[32]

This leaves the question of what this principle is. Ascribing agency to a living body seems highly problematic. In the *Essay*, Locke says that no idea of the beginning of motion can be drawn from bodies. *Contra* More, the instance of the billiard balls is intended to show that alterations are transferred in bodies without affording any idea of their original production.[33] When, in the letter addressed to Thomas Molyneux dated the 20th

---

[31] Kenneth Dewhurst, "Locke and Sydenham on the Teaching of Anatomy," *Medical History*, 2 (1958), 1-12; John R. Milton, "Locke, Medicine and the Mechanical Philosophy," *British Journal for the History of Philosophy*, 9 (2001), 221-43; Guy G. Meynell, "John Locke and the Preface to Thomas Sydenham's *Observationes Medicae*," *Medical History*, 50 (2006), 93–110,"

[32] Ephraïm Chambers, *Cyclopedia, or An Universal Dictionary of Arts and Sciences*, 2 vols. (London, 1728); 2 supplements vols. 1753), vol.1, s.v. "Faculty," 5.

[33] Henry More had said in his "Responsio ad fragmentum Cartesii" to Claude Clerselier (July-August 1655) that Descartes was "fabricating some kind of life when two bodies meet" "since no motion passes from one body into another, it is manifest that one arouses the other from sleep as it were, and in this way aroused bodies transfer themselves from place to place by their own force, which property of bodies I consider as

of January, 1693, Locke enjoins him to avoid "hypothesis taken from gra-
tis" and to discover the "natural functions of body" by observation; he
does not refer to any agency of the body—probably because there is no
need to, in his view.[34] In physics, the manifest cause merely has to be
pointed out, from an external point of view, by observation and analogy.
The experimental model inspires a methodology where the physician is
external to the observed phenomenon, so that the alleged powers that
can explain it are not active powers (known by reflection) but only passive ones; i.e., powers which "continue alteration" and do not impel motion.

This is the point: for Whytt, the constant renewal of respiration and
circulation cannot be physiologically explained other than by the perpetual exertion of the active power. It certainly remains puzzling how
this living subject (which is not the living body, but only operates in it,
through it and by its means) can be conceived of as continuing to exist
in a dead body—and particularly in excised muscles. Some clarification
is provided, in the third edition of the *Essay*, by the discussion of Porter-
field's theory, which Whytt holds as a variant of Stahl's theses. Whytt
criticizes their position for two reasons: firstly, identifying the active principle with a *logos* (rationally and voluntarily operating at the beginning
of life, and then being habitually exerted) is not supported by experimental evidence; secondly, accounting for the physiological motions in the
living body and the dead body by different principles is illogical. In the
same way, in the polemic with Haller, he will use this latter point to coun-
ter the mechanical account of irritation: as the physiological phenomena
in living bodies are only explained by the intervention of the active principle, these phenomena in dead bodies must be explained by the same
cause. The physiological phenomena must be of the same nature,
whether the body in which they take place be dead or excised, or

---

some shadow and image of life" (quoted by Henry in "Occult Qualities," 336). See also
Nicolas Malebranche, *The Search after Truth*, trans., Thomas M. Lennon and Paul J.
Olscamp (Cambridge, 1997), III.ii.3, VI.ii.3 and XVth Eclaircissement. David Hume,
Enquiry concerning Human Understanding, in Lewis A. Selby-Bigge, ed., rev. by Peter H.
Nidditch, *Hume's Enquiries*, 3rd ed. (Oxford, 1975); Tom L. Beauchamp, ed. (Oxford, 1999),
sections IV-V.
[34] *The Correspondence of John Locke*, ed., Esmond S. de Beer, 8 vols. (Oxford, 1981), let-
ter n. 1593.

decerebrated, or normally alive. Remarkably, there is no demarcation between the natural study of passive powers and the metaphysical or theological study of active powers in Whytt's philosophy. For instance, Thomas Reid will famously advance such a demarcation between physic and metaphysic in his letter to Henry Home Lord Kames dated the 16th of December, 1780, though in his physiological lectures he will agree with Whytt that materialism fails to study living bodies.[35] But Whytt employs the notion of active power *in* the physiological explanation, due to the particular nature of the medical object.

In addition to the physiological arguments, let us now look for any metaphysical justification. Wright points out that Whytt's physiology presupposes a kind of "substance dualism." Indeed, Whytt explicitly says that the living principle "is not distinct from the soul." But his use of the word 'substance' is ambiguous. In the text quoted above, he qualifies the agent as subject or being rather than as substance. In the introduction, the mind is said to act on the muscles by means of the "substance in the nerves":

> Although we may be at a loss to explain the nature of that substance in the nerves, by whose intervention the mind seems to act upon the muscles; and though we may be unacquainted with the intimate structure of those fibres upon which this substance operates, yet we have no room to doubt that voluntary motion is produced by the immediate energy of the mind ; manifold experience convincing us, that though there be required certain conditions in the body in order to its performance, it is nevertheless owing to the will. Nor ought we to be surprised when we meet with these kind of difficulties; for they attend most of our inquiries and researches.—Thus, though the laws of motion and gravitation be fully understood and demonstrated by philosophers, yet the first cause of motion the manner in which it is communicated to bodies, and the nature of gravity itself have never been explained.[36]

Strictly speaking, the active living principle alone is the living thing. Whytt feels justified in assuming an active sentient being because he does not attribute life to inert matter. Moreover, he does not presuppose that the physiological thing or *res vivens* is a substance in which another

---

[35] *The Correspondence of Thomas Reid*, ed., Paul Wood (University Park, PA and Edinburgh, 2002), 142 ; *Animate Creation*, 122-23.
[36] Whytt, *Essay*, 2-3.

agent operates, because for him, this thing is none other than the agent. The consequence of this is clear: matter endowed with passive powers is not one of the substantial components of the *res vivens*. Material arrangement is only the occasion for as well as the condition and object of the exertion of the immaterial power. Basically, he wishes to sustain a causal dualism in which agency, on the one hand, and mechanical connections, on the other, are distinguished.[37] But he does not take pains to demonstrate any substantial knowledge. He is only concerned with arguing that life is an experience of an active power and, as such, has to be accounted for as an effect of an agency. For this reason, he thinks that the notion of power involved in physiology is closer to voluntary power than to any so-called "action" of inert bodies. Certainly, in the text above, the assertion of a substance of nerves distinct from the mind seems questionable. Yet, in the light of Whytt's experimental evidence, it could be concluded that the substance in the nerves is the immaterial principle exerting itself via the occasion offered by the nerves. What is puzzling cannot be the immateriality of the living principle, but the substantiality of the mind. Mind, rather than living principle, seems to be a substance within a substance. Indeed, if the subject is the living being, it would be more appropriate to conceive of the mind as a mere faculty of this being (a faculty in the Lockean sense; i.e., an ability, not an agent). But it seems that, in 1751, this approach was off limits. Anyway, as the quotation shows, Whytt seems to agree with Hume in saying that we have no knowledge of the connection between the energy of the mind in the nerves, and the muscular motions.[38]

From a Humean Point of View

In the same year, 1751, Hume published the *Philosophical Essays* in a new edition, entitled *An Enquiry concerning Human Understanding*, together with *An Enquiry concerning the Principles of Morals*. In the seventh section of the first *Enquiry*, he offered strong arguments against any attempt to derive the idea of power from "an impression" either of sensation or

---

[37] If so, such a causal dualism is altogether different from the "function dualism" that Wright pointed out in La Mettrie's and Cullen's thought.

[38] Whytt, *Essay*, introduction, 2-3.

of reflection. His main target was John Locke, who in the chapter "Of power" argued, as seen above, that we get the notion of power from the experience of will and of the perception of ideas. Strictly speaking, the alleged powers exerted in the physiological motions were not the main object of the debate; however, Hume claimed "that our idea of power is not copied from any sentiment or consciousness of power within ourselves, when we give rise to animal motion, or apply our limbs to their proper use and office."[39] As we have just seen, the introduction to Whytt's *Essay* takes the exact opposite position to that of Hume, inferring the possibility of a connection between mind and motion in the case of organic motions from the experience of this connection in respect to voluntary motions. Whytt, while he acknowledges that we cannot know how this connection is performed, nevertheless insists that our experience clearly establishes that some motions are "owing to the will."

Hume's argument is put forward in the discussion on the thesis that the notion of connective power is obtained via the experience of the will as cause. Notably, Hume acknowledges that we feel the mind's determination to move on from an impression to another idea, but he contests any suggestion that this forceful feeling might constitute a consciousness of an ontological connection between a cause and an effect. In order to prove that we have no awareness of the connection between will and motion, he proceeds in three steps. First, he interprets the substantial dualism by means of his own principle of conceivability, in order to subvert the notion of power that Descartes himself put forward: we conceive of the soul clearly and distinctly without any need to conceive of the body, as we may conceive of the motion of one billiard ball moving in a straight line toward another independently of the motion of the latter. Then, Hume stresses that we cannot provide any reason why the will should be a power felt in some parts of the body and not in the others. Thus, the distinction between voluntary and involuntary motions is puzzling for Hume, who wonders "why has the will an influence over the tongue and fingers, not over the heart and liver?" The only source of certainty we can have in these questions is habit. Lastly, Hume assumed as an uncontroversial fact that voluntary motions involve physiological motions, which are neither conscious nor felt:

---

[39] Hume, *Enquiry*, VII.i, SB 67, 139.

> We learn from anatomy, that the immediate object of power in voluntary motion, is not the member itself which is moved, but certain muscles, and nerves, and animal spirits, and perhaps, something still more minute and more unknown, through which the motion is successively propagated, ere it reach the member itself whose motion is the immediate object of volition.[40]

Though Hume seems to endorse mechanistic anatomy, the model probably includes any anatomist explanation arising from the Boerhaavean framework, quite possibly including, in later editions, Whytt's. Yet Hume's and Whytt's intentions are quite contradictory. Hume uses the reference to anatomical inquiries to prove that claiming to experience the power of the will over the body is playing with words. Hume does not hold that the anatomist and the physiologist know the connection between will and muscular effect by any direct acquaintance with it. Indeed, in the second part of the seventeenth section, he shows that the scientific supposition of powers stems only from the observation of a constant conjunction.[41] But here, Hume only needs to show that the corporeal facts which follow any volition are quite unperceived, and that the motion we feel, coming at the end of the chain of so-called effects, is remote from the activating will. Conversely, observing conjunctions between motions and feelings which cannot be mechanistically explained, Whytt accepts a connection between physiological motions and agency. As seen above, no observation can define *how* the connection operates. We only know this connection as an unquestionable fact, according to Whytt. A mechanistic account cannot be drawn from the observation of a conjunction between feeling (e.g., the uneasiness prior to inspiration) and involuntary motion (e.g., of the intercostal muscles), probably because this conjunction is evidence of a causality that would be described nowadays as "known without observation," for it is proprioceptive.[42] For Whytt, experience is the standard not only for observed facts, but also for felt ones. Actually, Hume too admits that for the science of human nature, experience is a standard in this sense (i.e., felt as well as observed). For instance, belief and passion are felt in myself as well as observed in other people. In the introduction to the *Treatise*, Hume seems to argue that only the

---

[40]   *Ibid.*, VII.i SB 66, 138.
[41]   Hume, *Enquiry*, VII.ii SB 74-75, 144.
[42]   Gertrude Elizabeth Margaret Anscombe, *Intention* (Oxford, 1957, 1963), § 8-10.

moral philosopher (inquiring into human nature) needs to observe spontaneous experiments which cannot be premeditated or purposely construed. In the other natural sciences, causal inferences are drawn from mere observed conjunctions.[43] The case of Whytt's physiology seems to complicate this division; let's consider its epistemological basis in Humean terms.

A power is only believed in because we feel vividly, lively, strongly the idea (e.g., the fire) that is associated with a present impression (e.g., smoke). This mental force is acquired through the habitual observation of past conjunctions (e.g., between fire and smoke). Remarkably, for Hume, ignorance of the circumstance by which an alleged cause is cause does not preclude belief in the cause. Moreover the inference of an energy from experience and feeling is not rejected by Hume. He goes on to speak of "energy of the mind" accounting for the forceful belief in powers, though this energy cannot be taken for a "connection" between some mental act and some bodily effect. To Hume, as to Hutcheson, a feeling is an original fact, phenomenally described. We cannot know if the force of belief is not, as such, a connective power; but such is our constitution that we cannot avoid taking it as an "energy" or as an effect of power. This belief about the condition of any belief is an original fact of our nature. Later, in the *Dialogue concerning Religion*, the sceptic Philo will acknowledge the natural belief that "the rotting of a turnip, the generation of an animal, and *the structure of human thought*" are "energies that probably bear some remote analogy to each other." But Hume will not attempt to explore the assumption of those living energies.[44] In the *Enquiry*, it is said that the believed power depends on the kind of causality by which our perceptions are linked. If the association of causality is "direct," we observe first one fact, then another, taking the first as a cause and the second as an effect. If the causality is "collateral," we find by experience that two facts are conjoined and we conceive that they are caused by a common power. Whytt's assumptions could be seen as natural inferences

---

[43] David Hume, *A Treatise of Human Nature*, ed,. Lewis A. Selby-Bigge, rev. by Peter H. Nidditch (Oxford, 1975); ed., David F. Norton and Mary J. Norton (Cambridge, 2007), 5-6.
[44] Hume's use of animal aeconomy in the arguments of the Dialogue concerning Natural Religion has been documented by Rivers, "'Galen's Muscles'" and Peter Knox-Shaw, "Hume's 'farther scenes': Maupertuis and Buffon in the *Dialogues*," *Hume Studies*, 34 (2008), 209-30.

from feeling, either direct or collateral. We have seen that Whytt denies any knowledge of the connection between mind-energy in the nerves and the muscles; however, he assumes that there is experimental evidence of the energy of the mind in the nerves, including the feeling of the organs. This proves the existence of the power, because only an agent can feel the stimulus which will lead to material, unexpected effects.[45] The collateral action of sympathy is another piece of evidence. For Whytt, feeling is an original fact (included in the phenomenon of sympathy) whose subject is the living principle, which in turn is the only possible cause of the consequences. The role of feeling is to determine the quantity of energy to provide.[46] So the exertion of the active principle in motion is matched to the irritation felt—in a way that we cannot explain. But according to Whytt the feeling is itself an action of the living principle. Because Whytt conceives of sensibility as a physiological function, he is forced to consider feeling itself as an affective experience of the power invested in the nerves. Thus, he takes the nervous conditions associated with exertion of the power of feeling as originally inseparable (by virtue of our constitution) from this power. In contrast, Hume's concern with physiology is very limited because the fundamental level from which the science of human nature must proceed is the experience of our mental operations (beliefs and passions)—as a psychological experience phenomenally described. In Hume's view, a physiological explanation, while ensuring some degree of accuracy in the observation, would also introduce an external point of view that would leave no room for the

---

[45] The assumption of active principles from experience was sustained in the articles of Henry Home and John Stewart which were published along with two articles by Stewart in the first volume of the *Essays and Observations Physical and Literary*, edited by Monro and Hume and published in 1754. Home and Stewart take for granted that experience gives us evidence that moving (e.g. walking) and communicating motion (e.g. moving other things) imply the exercise of active powers. But Home thought that active principles were inherent to matter whereas Stewart defended that matter cannot begin motion and "active beings" only are immaterial self-movers. Henry Home, "Of the Laws of Motion," and John Stewart, "Some Remarks on the Laws of Motion, and the Intertia of Matter," in *Essays and Observations, Physical and Literary*, ed. A Monro (Edinburgh, 1754).

[46] On such a presupposition, being admitted that matter is passive and that action of human active beings is accompanied by the consciousness of passion, see for instance Stewart, "Laws of Motions," 73-74.

phenomenal one.[47] And yet, as we have seen, Whytt's observations include reference to feeling as phenomenally grasped.

Towards a Milder Immaterialism

Whytt endeavoured to conceive of a living agency without any endorsement of the substantial form, and to offer the experience of energy as a physiological explanation, without claiming to understand *how* the connection (either direct, for instance between irritation and contraction of an excised muscle; or collateral, for instance between different organs in sympathy) works. Yet it is not clear that he found this entirely satisfactory. In the later *Observations on the Nature, Cause, and Cure of those Disorders which have been commonly called Nervous, Hyponcondriac or Hysteric*, first published in 1764, he assumes in the first chapter "on the structure, the use and the sympathy of the nerves" that they "communicate sense and a power of motion to body," although we do not know whether or not the fluid that circulates in them is *a medium* through which they accomplish their actions.[48] In fact, in this work, Whytt proves to be very cautious on metaphysical issues: he does not refer explicitly to the "immaterial principle," but only to a "sentient power of the nerves." In comparison to 1751, the increasing importance of the nerves as organs of sensibility is striking. Surprisingly, the expression "the agency of the nerves" is employed, probably to stress their crucial role.[49] Whereas, in the *Essay*, the stimulus was not an explanation for all involuntary mo-

---

[47] In the *Treatise*, Hume has recourse to "an imaginary dissection of the brain" only once, in order to account for the mistakes that arise from resemblance, contiguity and causation: "the animal spirits run into all the contiguous traces and rouze up the other ideas, that are related to [a given conception]" (*Treatise*, SB 60, 44). Contrary to the physiological explanation, the description of belief in terms of *perceptions* (impressions and ideas) is an attempt to capture the phenomenal experience with respect to "vivacity."

[48] Robert Whytt, *Observations on the Nature, Cause, and Cure of those Disorders which have been commonly called Nervous, Hyponcondriac or Hysteric, To Which are Prefixed Some Remarks on the Sympathy of the Nerves* (Edinburgh, [1764] 1765), 3.

[49] Whytt, *Observation*, 3 and 203. Whytt might have been prepared for softening his immaterialism by his chemical and pharmacological inquiries. The defence of active principles inherent to matter was frequently founded on this chemical evidence. For instance, see Henry Home, "Laws of motion," 10.

tions (but only for alternating muscular motions), Whytt claims in 1764: "There are only two kinds of motion observed in the bodies of living animals, *viz.* voluntary, and involuntary from *stimuli*."[50] He highlights the role of sympathy or consent of the parts thanks to which the motion from stimulus "continues for some time, tho' in a much weaker degree, even in those muscles, whose connection with the brain is wholly cut off." Incidentally, the immaterialism here seems milder. Notwithstanding, the other causes are still described as only "occasioning" their effect. And, more importantly, the *subjective* notions of feeling and sympathy still preclude any mechanical account.[51] This is the reason why, even though he cautiously avoids any metaphysical commitment in this work, Whytt maintains the assumption of an active power with which the living being is identified. The nerves perform an action whose origin is not their material structure, but implicitly is the "living principle." While we might regret that such an agency is not more accurately defined,[52] in Whytt's

---

[50] Whytt, *Observations*, ch. 1. The role of stimulus became the key to understanding diseases whose symptoms are not nervous, such as fevers or croup. Whytt, *Manuscripts*, MS. 6863 and 6865.

[51] Whytt, *Observations*, 32: "Could we suppose the circulation of the blood were to remain, after a total abolition of the sentient powers of the brain and nerves, there would be no more sympathy between the parts of such an animal body, than between those any hydraulic machine. As in this case, the motion of the fluids would be merely mechanical, so every change made in any parts, must be the result of mechanism alone, and consequently very different from consent, which, as it depends upon feeling, cannot be explained upon mechanical principles." See Whytt, *Observations*, 501.

[52] John Pringle (M.D., F.R.S.) expressed to Robert Whytt this very regret. In a letter dated April 21st, 1759, Pringle appears dissatisfied with Whytt's description. He gives Whytt advice on some "sheet of [his papers]" (probably an early draft of the *Observations on Nervous Diseases*): "As to general, I still think that your work will appear lame without the addition of a part upon the consensus partum. Indeed I do not think that you shall prove those symptoms you call hysteria and hypocondria to be more nervous, than fibrous or vascular or what you will. Consider that the consent of parts has been hitherto [*illegible*] by the systematics in a very vague and abstruse manner, some restricting it to the nerves only, others extending it to the blood, vessels, membranes &c. Tho' a medical writer is not always obliged to precise the anatomy or physiology of the parts that are the seat of the disease he treats of, yet to be sure, if the structure is not generally understood and if the action of the parts are [*illegible*] it behaves the author to tell at least what kind of principles relating to those parts he adopts" (Whytt, *Manuscripts*, MS 6867/1/1/2/1). In an undated letter, he says again "In the first place, he [the reader] does not know what you mean by nervous symptoms, 2ndly he does not well know what

view the main point is probably settled: in physiological accounts, the agency referred to is internal and experienced by the living subject. Whytt uses the word "consent" to mean the corporeal whole and chooses "sympathy" to denote that "by means of which many operations are carried on in sound state." Implicitly, why any irritation might be painful can be explained by its being in conflict with a healthy state in normal cases, but at a deeper level, the intensity and the nature of the ailment depend on "the greater or lesser natural delicacy or sensibility of the patient's nerves."[53] This disorder is an original fact in the major pathological cases: it is a "predisposition." The nescient appeal to the constitution, traditional in the Scottish Enlightenment, is employed in a more individual sense. Thus, the nervous disorder which causes hysteria and hypochondria can be not only material ("a fault in the coats, the medullary substance or the fluid in the nerves") but also be due to the fact that "the sentient power of the nerves may be either too acute, obtuse, depraved, or wholly wanting," which produces disagreeable sensations, irregular motions or convulsions, wrong stimulations or a general weakness in different parts of the body. The cure consists in removing accidental or occasional causes if any; but when the cause is "in the constitution" or "original," the cure cannot be perfect. A disorder of sensibility thus constitutes a "depravation" in the power of life.

Thomas Reid, whose interest in physiology in general and in Whytt's studies in particular were documented by Paul Wood, was well aware of the difficulties attending the assumption of a sentient principle:

> For we feel nothing of this kind in the circulation of the blood the motion of the lungs or peristaltick motion of the gutts. And a stimulus that is not felt or perceived seems to border upon a contradiction. Or at least to signify only an unknown somewhat. Like an occult quality. Or will it be said that there is a sentient principle in us distinct from the mind which feels this stimulus and is affected by it. For

---

you meant by feeling & motion of the nerves, & lastly has not the smallest idea of the depraved feeling of the nerves" (Letter from John Pringle to Robert Whytt, April 21st, 1759, in Whytt, *Manuscripts*, MS 6867/1/1/2/3). Pringle became President of the Royal Society of Edinburgh in 1777.

53) Whytt, *Observations*, 164. In normal cases, sensibility would prompt motions "proportional only to the strength of body in general," and those motions "would be carried on in the manner most proper for the purposes of health" (Whytt, *Manuscripts*, MS 6878, Miscellaneous Notes, file 6, "Nervous Diseases").

I think it cannot with any propriety of language be said that mere inert matter is acted upon by a stimulus. Or perhaps it may be said that tho' the mind had in the beginning a perception of this stimulus yet like other feelings of pleasure and pain it becomes insensible by habits. But this last hypothesis labour<s> under this prejudice that it seems a general rule that where a stimulus by habit & use becomes insensible it loses its effect so those that sneeze upon taking snuff give over doing so when it comes to a habit.[54]

The power of a stimulus in organic and apparently insensible phenomena remains bizarre to Reid. Moreover, avoiding Locke's objection, he clearly dismisses the idea that this power can be ascribed to "a sentient principle in us distinct from the mind." He rules out any active principle inherent to matter too. His indebtedness to Locke leads him to define active power as "every thing that incites us to act," leaving aside the question of whether there are such causes in animal oeconomy.[55] Finally, in 1795, in a late discourse entitled "Of muscular motions in the Human Body," he deals instead with a nervous power which, though we are at a loss to explain it, we have no reason to attribute to any subject other than our constitution. This is because the sole task of the naturalist is to point out general laws of nature according to which, when we want to do something, a nervous power is exerted and causes muscular motions. Reid claims here that occasionalism is of no recourse. There is a power, endowed in the nerves, which by a law of our natural constitution has certain effects. Indeed we remain "ignorant of our Frame and Make."[56] Whytt's superaddition of an immaterial principle appears now superfluous. The *constitution* is the sole living being.

To sum up, at the time Whytt was developing his theories, empiricist philosophy was already criticizing several aspects of the medical use of the notion of power. Indeed, the particular types of evidence that he finds constituted a challenge to the philosophy of the mind of the British Enlightenment. Whytt's experimentalism leads him to sidestep the main objections of philosophical empiricism and to take a new look at animation, treating it as an active power. It has become necessary to give caus-

---

[54] Thomas Reid, MS. 2131/7/II/2,1v, in Thomas Reid, *On the Animate Creation*, ed., Paul Wood (University Park, PA and Edinburgh, 1995), 102-103.

[55] Thomas Reid, *Essays on the Active Powers of Man*, ed., Knud Haakonssen (Edinburgh, 2010), I.vi.

[56] Reid, *Animate Creation*, 120.

al explanations of unexpected links between things in which cause and effect are not proportionate. Moreover, echoing Hutcheson who regarded 'passions' as "facts of our nature," Whytt refers to 'feeling' as the original experience of the power of life. In this respect, he bases himself on the conceptions of "active power" and "original fact" of the Scottish experimental theism. At some stage in his work, Whytt took for granted the immateriality of power. Yet another direction was later pointed out. Dr William Cullen, as Wright showed, did not hold the same metaphysical principles. Cullen was of the opinion that medicine deals with the mind-body problem only insofar as examining *how* one bodily state or part can affect another bodily state or part implies explaining how one state of the brain or the mind can affect another organ (such as the heart, for instance). Thus, the power of the soul is no longer the *explanans*, but becomes the *explanandum*. For Cullen does not suppose that the mind-body union explains physiological phenomena by an immaterial agency. It is the physiological inquiry which accounts for the natural fact that is the action of the mind or brain on the body. With this new metaphysics in hand, Cullen seems ready for another shift. The original fact in medicine is no longer animation, but the organisation of the bodily system in which different levels of causality are involved.[57]

---

[57] My thanks go to Marjorie Sweetko for her careful reading. This work was supported by a grant from French National Research Agency (Project ANR-09-JCJC -0145-01, "Philomed – La refonte de l'homme").

II. ARTS OF EMPIRICAL RESEARCH

Learning to Read Nature:
Francis Bacon's Notion of Experiential Literacy
(*Experientia Literata*)

Guido Giglioni

*The Warburg Institute**

Abstract

Francis Bacon's elusive notion of experience can be better understood when we relate it to his views on matter, motion, appetite and intellect, and bring to the fore its broader philosophical implications. Bacon's theory of knowledge is embedded in a programme of disciplinary redefinition, outlined in the *Advancement of Learning* and *De augmentis scientiarum*. Among all disciplines, *prima philosophia* (and not *metaphysica*) plays a key foundational role, based on the idea of both a *physical* parallelism between the human intellect and nature (psycho-physical parallelism) and a *theological* parallelism between nature and God (physico-theological parallelism). Failure to assess Bacon's distinctive position concerning the way in which the mind mirrors both the natural and the divine world, that is to say, the meaning of "reality," has resulted in notoriously jejune discussions on Baconian empiricism, monotonously driven by epistemological concerns. As a result, the standard view on Bacon's empiricism is as epistemologically comforting as it is imaginary, an "idol" in a genuinely Baconian sense. In this article, Bacon's notion of experience will be discussed by examining those steps that he considered to be the crucial initial stages in the formation of human experience, stages described as a process of experiential literacy (*experientia literata*) or, in emblematic terms, as a hunting expedition led by the mythological figure of Pan (*venatio Panis*). I argue that a well-rounded analysis of Bacon's *experientia literata* needs to take into account the complementary notion of the "spelling-book of nature" (*abecedarium naturae*), that is, the original code of the primordial motions of matter. By getting acquainted with the first rudiments of

* The Warburg Institute, School of Advanced Study, University of London, Woburn Square, London, WC1H 0AB (guido.giglioni@sas.ac.uk). Research leading to this article was supported by the ERC Grant 241125 MOM ('The Medicine of the Mind and Natural Philosophy in Early Modern England: A New Way of Interpreting Francis Bacon'). Translations from Bacon's Latin works are mine. I would like to thank an anonymous reader for his comments and suggestions.

experience through its spelling-book (on both an individual and a cosmological level), one learns to read the book of nature and, most of all, to write new pages in it.

Keywords
experiential literacy, *experientia literata*, Pan's hunt, nature, matter, physics, metaphysics

1. Introduction

Despite the apparently anodyne simplicity of such notions as "induction" and "experience," Francis Bacon's theory of knowledge presents an extremely complex account of the processes that define the activity of the human mind. It assumes that mankind can achieve a condition of thorough transparency between the intellect (*mens*) and reality (*res*) once a series of precautions, preparations and prerequisites are fulfilled. In the state of cognitive purity prior to the Fall, the mind was able to mirror reality, and this condition will return to be the norm once the mind will be reconciled with nature at the end of the great restoration of being (*instauratio magna*). In the meantime, in the current situation of post-lapsarian disgrace, human beings can rely on cognitive apparatuses (the senses—external and internal—and the intellect) and on mechanisms of acquisition and accumulation of knowledge which by and large are able to provide a reliable representation of reality.

Regardless of all post-lapsarian interferences and distortions, Bacon is convinced that a form of ontological parallelism still applies between matter and the intellect: everything that occurs in the sphere of matter (*globus materiae*) is reflected in the sphere of the intellect (*globus intellectus*).[1] Among other things, this ontological parallelism allows Bacon to present the disciplinary divisions (*partitiones*) through which he articulates his system of knowledge as corresponding to the very reality

---

[1] On the ontological parallelism between matter and intellect, see Francis Bacon, *De augmentis scientiarum*, in *Works*, eds. James Spedding, Robert L. Ellis, D.D. Heath, 14 vols. (London, 1857–1874; repr. Stuttgart-Bad Cannstatt, 1962; Cambridge, 2012), I, 772. See also *Redargutio philosophiarum*, about the relationship between *globus materiatus* and *globus intellectualis* (*Works*, III, 584), and *Cogitata et visa*, about the relationship between the *novus orbis scientiarum* and the *novus orbis terrarum* (*Works*, III, 612). In fact, since the book of nature mirrors the sacred scriptures, the parallelism between nature and the mind is based on a deeper physico-theological parallelism. This aspect in Bacon's metaphysics will not be discussed in this article.

of things and not as arbitrary distinctions devised by the mind.[2] According to the principles of Bacon's metaphysics, matter is pervaded by a clearly defined set of primordial appetites, which manifest themselves in the form of tendencies and perceptions (*perceptiones*).[3] These perceptions are at the origin of both the forms that make up all natural phenomena and every process of knowledge in nature, from animal sensations to human intellections. As a result of the ontological parallelism between matter and the intellect, just as reality evolves from original appetites to sensible particulars and then structural forms, so knowledge ascends from material perceptions to sensations and then axioms.[4] Bacon describes with meticulous attention all the steps through which the human mind adjusts itself to reality, in a progression of increasing accuracy and faithfulness: *sylva* (or *materies, supellex, farrago, massa*), *experientia illiterata, experientia literata, historia, topica particularis, glossa prima*—or *paraphrasis*—*circa interpretationem naturae, interpretatio naturae, inductio, philosophia prima, physica* and *metaphysica*. The transition from *sylva* to *metaphysica* coincides with the process through which the mind corresponds to the reality of things. In this process, cognitive literacy—*experientia literata*—plays a crucial role. The subject of this article is the notion of *experientia literata*.[5]

---

[2] Bacon, *De augmentis scientiarum*, in *Works*, I, 540.

[3] On Bacon's notion of material motion as appetite, see *Novum organum*, in *The* Instauratio Magna *Part II*: Novum Organum *and Associated Texts*, eds. Graham Rees and Maria Wakely (Oxford, 2004), Oxford Francis Bacon [henceforth abbreviated as OFB], XI, 382; *Cogitationes de natura rerum*, in *Works*, III, 22; *Sylva Sylvarum*, in *Works*, II, 618-19. On the difference between *perceptio* and *sensus*, see *De augmentis scientiarum*, in *Works*, I, 610-11; *Sylva Sylvarum*, in *Works*, II, 603.

[4] Significantly, Bacon's uses the horns of Pan to give an emblematic representation of the way forms result from the contraction of particulars into specific units. See *De sapientia veterum*, in *Works*, VI, 637: "Quod vero cornua hujusmodi ab imo latiora ad verticem acuta sint; id eo spectat, quod omnis rerum natura instar pyramidis acuta sit: individua enim infinita sunt; ea colliguntur in species et ipsas multiplices; species rursus insurgunt in genera; atque haec quoque ascendendo in magis generalia contrahuntur, ut tandem natura tanquam in unum coire videatur. Neque mirum est Panis cornua etiam coelum ferire; cum summitates naturae sive ideae universales etiam ad divina quodammodo pertingant. Paratus enim et propinquus est transitus a metaphysica ad theologiam naturalem."

[5] On *experientia literata*, see: Lisa Jardine, *Francis Bacon: Discovery and the Art of Discourse* (Cambridge, 1974), 143-49; eadem, "*Experientia Literata* or *Novum Organum*? The

Seen as a cultural phenomenon, Bacon's empiricism represents a fascinating chapter in the history of ideas. One wonders whether the difficulties that interpreters of his philosophy encounter today when they examine the notion of Baconian empiricism have to do with ideological and nationalistic biases, or simply with an incident in philosophical historiography, more than with actual exegetical obscurities in Bacon's texts. Generally speaking, if by "empiricism" one means a philosophical stance according to which human knowledge can only proceed from items that are provided by sense perception, we could say that Bacon elaborated and defended an original view concerning empiricism. By contrast, if by "empiricism" one means an ontological position according to which reality is in itself unknowable and what we know of things are only appearances mediated by our senses, then Bacon cannot, strictly speaking, be considered an empiricist, for, as I am going to argue in this article, he maintains that, beyond sense perceptions, the human mind has access— qualified as it may be—to structural aspects of reality, which he calls "forms" or "schematisms." By *forms*, Bacon means a definite number of dynamic arrangements of matter (veritable laws), through which matter is constantly being organized following specific patterns of an appetitive nature. Bacon's realist empiricism has been read taking Boyle's, Locke's and Hume's varieties of post-Cartesian empiricism as the hermeneutical norm, and, in an uncritical and dogmatic manner, it has been introduced as such into a certain self-interpretative tradition of philosophy, from Immanuel Kant to Karl Popper.[6]

Dilemma of Bacon's Scientific Method," in William A. Sessions, ed., *Francis Bacon's Legacy of Texts* (New York, 1990), 47-67; Marta Fattori, "*Experientia—experimentum*: Un confronto tra il corpus latino e inglese di Francis Bacon," in Marco Veneziani, ed., *Experientia* (Florence, 2002), 243-68; Cesare Pastorino, "Weighing Experience: Experimental Histories and Francis Bacon's Quantitative Program," *Early Science and Medicine*, 16 (2011), 542-70; Dana Jalobeanu, "Core Experiments, Natural Histories and the Art of *Experientia Literata*: The Meaning of Baconian Experimentation," *Societate şi Politică*, 5 (2011), 88-103; Laura Georgescu, "A New Form of Knowledge: *Experientia Literata*," *Societate şi Politică*, 5 (2011), 104-20; Ian G. Stewart, "*Res, veluti per Machinas, Conficiatur*: Natural History and the 'Mechanical' Reform of Natural Philosophy," *Early Science and Medicine*, 17 (2012), 87-111; Laura Georgescu and Mădălina Giurgea, "Redefining the Role of Experiment in Bacon's Natural History: How Baconian was Descartes before Emerging from His Cocoon?," *Early Science and Medicine*, 17 (2012), 158-180.

[6] I have examined this aspect of Bacon's *fortuna*, especially in its earliest phases, in

A second historiographic accident concerns the way in which Bacon's nuanced and multifaceted empiricism has been reduced to an example of inductive platitude. In this case, too, the textual situation is much more complicated than one might think. Bacon is extremely severe against all natural philosophical programmes in which experience is left to itself, as much as he is critical of the intellect when it is abandoned to its own devices (its idols). In his opinion, the domain of raw experience—"illiterate" experience—is *barren, superstitious* and *obsessive*. William Gilbert (1544–1603), the great investigator of magnetism, admired by Bacon for the remarkable results achieved through his meticulous investigations, is nevertheless also presented as the embodiment of an uncritical acceptance of experience, not illumined by far-reaching theoretical assumptions, in which the experimental attitude towards nature turns into an obsessive search after empirical particulars *qua* particulars. In the end, as Bacon writes in the *Novum organum*, Gilbert morphed into an actual loadstone, such was his inability to draw his attention away from phenomena other than magnetic.[7] This also means that a constructivist notion of knowledge can only plunge one's mind into forms of alienation from reality. In Bacon's opinion, reality is not what we make of it (both experimentally and mechanically), but what allows our knowledge to be translated into real action. *Materia, natura* e *res* pre-exist and define the possibilities and limits of human knowledge. In this sense, Bacon's theory of experience cannot be correctly understood when it is severed from its foundation in ontological realism.

Bacon refers to several metaphorical contexts to illustrate the process through which human beings accumulate experience (from purely accidental discoveries to investigations by deliberate trial and error, up to increasingly more sophisticated procedures to catalogue and interpret natural phenomena). These are: hunting, husbandry, gardening, shepherding, animal breeding, travelling, getting oriented in a forest, groping about in the dark, digesting food, but above all, learning to read and write. This last image, in particular, is what Bacon has in mind when he

---

"How Bacon Became Baconian," in Daniel Garber and Sophie Roux, eds., *The Mechanization of Natural Philosophy* (Dordrecht, 2013), 27-54.

[7] Bacon, *Novum organum*, in OFB, XI, 88, 100, 110. See also *Redargutio philosophiarum*, in *Works*, III, 571, and *Cogitata e visa*, in *ibid.*, 603.

suggests the idea of *experientia literata*, i.e., "cognitive literacy." Therefore, when in the *Advancement of Learning* and *De augmentis scientiarum* he introduces the distinction between *experientia illiterata* and *literata*, his intention is not to establish a difference between *unlearned* and *learned* empiricism (in line with the distinction recurrent at the time between natural history based on mechanical arts and humanistic natural history, or today in line with the distinction *à la mode académique* between vernacular and elitist knowledge). Rather, and much more simply, the dichotomy of illiterate and literate *experientia* follows Bacon's distinction between a level of unmediated experience, entirely engulfed in the life of nature, and a level of mediated experience, in which sense knowledge (*sensus*) begins to disentangle itself from the *sylva* of natural perceptions and appetites (*perceptio, appetitus, conatus, nisus*). While in the former stage, matter's *perceptiones* and the soul's *sensationes* are still unable to reach a degree of awareness, in the latter they rely on the first rudiments of experience and acquire a basic knowledge of the "alphabet of nature," so that the mind is able to have a first glimpse of nature's operations. In *Temporis partus masculus*, for instance, Hippocrates is criticised for being dazzled by natural phenomena, unable to raise his mind to the level of empirical literacy.[8] In sum, the difference between *experientia illiterata* and *experientia literata* is the difference between unmediated empiricism and empirical awareness.

In Bacon's view, as I will show in the course of this article, the rudiments of cognitive literacy represent the original ways in which we make experience of reality (*modi experimentandi*), where the word *experimentum* is to be taken in the general sense of "test," "attempt," "endeavour." *Experimentum* is the way in which a series of material circumstances are set up in order to have first-hand experience of specific phenomena and to get acquainted with things. Bacon theorizes the notion of experiential literacy (*experientia literata*) in Book 5 of *De augmentis scientiarum*, where he also provides concrete instantiations of the process under dis-

---

[8] Bacon, *Temporis partus masculus*, in *Works*, III, 534: "Atque iste homo [Hippocrates] certe in experientiae obtutu perpetuo haerere videtur, verum oculis non natantibus et anquirentibus, sed stupidis et resolutis. Deinde a stupore visu parum recollecto, idola quaedam, non immania quidem illa theoriarum, sed elegantiora ista quae superficiem historiae circumstant, excipit."

cussion.[9] However, we can say that he devoted an entire work to show
the procedures of cognitive literacy. This work is the undeservedly ne-
glected *Sylva Sylvarum*, published posthumously in 1626. Here one can
observe the process of *experientia literata* in its very making.[10] In my account of cognitive literacy, I will first contextualize Bacon's notion of
cognitive literacy within the broader framework of his theory of knowledge. It will become apparent that Bacon's views on knowledge need to
be examined by taking into account their ontological underpinnings. As
already said, knowledge (*globus intellectus*) and reality (*globus materiae*)
mirror each other unequivocally (it is the human mind, especially when
entangled in the snares of self-knowledge, that is responsible for the
production of all sorts of idolatrous representations):

> the true norm for a legitimate inquiry is that *nothing is found in the sphere of mat-
> ter which does not have a parallel in the crystal sphere, that is, the intellect.*[11]

This ontological mirroring can be called a psycho-physical parallelism
between the intellect and matter.

2. Theory of Knowledge

Book 3 of *De augmentis scientiarum* contains a concise and cogent discussion of ideas concerning knowledge and metaphysics. Indeed, it can
be seen as a précis of Baconian ontology. Bacon's theory of knowledge,
as already outlined in the *Advancement of Learning*, presupposes three

---

[9] Bacon refers briefly to *experientia literata* in *Novum organum*, OFB XI, 158-160. In
Aphorism 101, Part 2, *experientia literata*, described as a form of *scriptio*, is contrasted
with *memoria* and *meditatio*, as faculties that do not rely on technological developments
(*ibid.*, 158).

[10] On this point, see Guido Giglioni, "Mastering the Appetites of Matter: Francis Bacon's
Sylva Sylvarum," in Charles T. Wolfe and Ofer Gal, eds., *The Body as Object and Instrument of Knowledge: Embodied Empiricism in Early Modern Science* (Dordrecht, 2010),
149-67. On *Sylva Sylvarum*, see David Colclough, "'The Materialls for the Building': Reu-
niting Francis Bacon's *Sylva Sylvarum* and *New Atlantis*," *Intellectual History Review*, 20
(2010), 181-200.

[11] Bacon, *De augmentis scientiarum*, in *Works*, I, 772: "*legitimae inquisitionis vera norma
est*, ut nihil inveniatur in globo materiae, quod non habeat parallelum in globo crystal-
lino sive intellectu."

levels of reality—description (*historia*, "history"), fiction (*poësis*, "poesy") and intellectual vision (*scientia*)—corresponding to three divisions of the human soul: memory, imagination and reason. Reason, *scientia* and intellectual vision represent the highest level of intimacy that the human mind can enjoy with things ("history" is too prostrate on the ground, "poesy" indulges in dreams). The process of knowledge, says Bacon at the beginning of Book 3, resembles the cycle of waters in nature: some of them "fall from the sky," some others "emanate from earth." Likewise, the sources of knowledge are to be found both here on earth (*hic infra*) and up there in heaven (*in alto*):

> Every knowledge (*scientia*) has two sources of information: the one is divinely inspired; the other derives from the senses.[12]

This means that *scientia* can be divided into theology and philosophy. Here theology has the strict and technical meaning of "inspired and sacred" theology, not "natural" theology, which is instead part of philosophy. *Scientia* can therefore come either directly from God or from the senses. When knowledge comes from the senses, its sources are three: God, nature and the soul (*philosophiae objectum triplex, Deus, Natura, Homo*). Here again, as in the case of inspired knowledge, God is seen by Bacon as a source of knowledge, but with the difference that this time He is mediated through the objects of the creation. God, nature and the human soul represent three ontological domains that, with respect to knowledge, are hierarchically ordered according to their power to "strike" the intellect:

> Nature strikes the intellect with *a direct ray*; God, because of an uneven medium (i.e., the creatures), strikes it with a *refracted ray*; man, insofar as he is shown and displayed to himself, strikes the intellect with a *reflected ray*.[13]

The optical image here used by Bacon is very eloquent. First and foremost, from the point of view of human knowledge, nature—more than God or the soul—is the direct and immediate object of the intellect (*na-*

---

[12] *Ibid.*, 539. The empiricist assumption that all knowledge derives from the senses does not apply in Bacon's metaphysics.

[13] *Ibid.*, 540.

tura percutit intellectum radio directo). Secondly, as already said, God can either be a supernatural source of knowledge (thoroughly transcendent and entirely unknowable), or an object of knowledge, mediated through the creation. Refractions of God through nature form the basis of natural theology. Self-knowledge, finally, is exposed to the many illusions and deceptions of self-reflexivity, for knowledge of nature as reflected in the soul is far more removed from the reality of things than direct knowledge of nature and knowledge of God through nature.

Natural theology as part of philosophy is "knowledge (*scientia*), or rather a spark of knowledge (*scientia*) as one can have of God through the light of nature (*lumen naturae*) and the contemplation of the created things."[14] Being mediated by the light of nature, natural theology is included in natural knowledge, with the difference that, within the sphere of natural philosophy, intellect and nature are on an ontological par, while in natural theology the intellect find itself in an asymmetrical relationship with God and therefore it needs to adapt itself to that superior object: "he who will try to adjust the celestial mysteries of religion to our reason will toil in vain. Rather, it will be more appropriate for our minds to raise themselves to worship the throne of the celestial truth."[15] As part of natural philosophy, natural theology can expand the range of knowledge provided by the *lumen naturae*, for the human mind can rely on "ascending" and "descending" ladders of knowledge.[16] For instance, apart from the Bible (*ex locis Scripturae Sacrae*), knowledge of angels and demons is possible either "through the ladder of corporeal things" (*ex experientia*) or through introspection (*ex ratione*), by examining one's soul (*in anima humana veluti in speculo*).[17]

One conclusion one can draw from this section of *De augmentis scientiarum* is that the reality and certainty of knowledge depend either on God's direct inspiration (*theologia sacra*) or on intellectual access to na-

---

[14] *Ibid.*, 544.

[15] *Ibid.*, 545.

[16] *Ibid.*, 547: "quandoquidem omnis solida et fructuosa naturalis philosophia duplicem adhibeat scalam, eamque diversam; *ascensoriam* et *descensoriam*; *ab experientia ad axiomata*, et *ab axiomatibus ad nova inventa*." On the religious meaning of the ascending and descending ladder, see also Bacon, *A Confession of Faith*, in *The Major Works*, ed. Brian Vickers (Oxford, 1996), 107.

[17] Bacon, *De augmentis scientiarum*, in *Works*, I, 546.

ture beginning with the senses. Natural theology and knowledge of the soul, however important and rich, are less reliable. Divine inspiration, on the other hand, despite being most certain, escapes human control by its very nature. *Philosophia* is therefore the field of knowledge that is entirely open to human inquiry. Depending on its three main objects (*Deus, Natura, Homo*), it can be further divided into three types of investigation (*doctrinae*): natural theology (*doctrina de numine*), natural philosophy (*doctrina de natura*) and human philosophy (*doctrina de homine*). These three principal subdivisions, however, are not "like different lines that converge into one angle;" rather, they are similar to "the branches which are joined in one trunk," a trunk, Bacon continues, that "up to a certain point is undivided and continuous, before splitting into branches." The image is worth keeping in mind: Bacon prefers the natural, real image of the tree, with its branches growing naturally and spontaneously out of common roots and one trunk, rather than the geometrical, constructivist image of lines forming angles. The trunk of the tree represents the common foundation of knowledge prior to all disciplinary divisions, the "universal science, which is the mother of all other sciences," the *philosophia prima,* also known as *sapientia,* "which once used to be defined as *knowledge of divine and human things*."[18] Here it is also crucial to point out that the disciplinary "partitions" are not arbitrary, for they correspond to real divisions of being. Bacon is firmly of the opinion that there is a metaphysical unity underlying human learning, a metaphysical unity which is also the rationale behind his attempt to reorganize and reform human knowledge in *De augmentis scientiarum.* Such a project, Bacon confirms in Book 4, cannot produce any artificial break within the seamless process of knowledge (*solutio continuitatis in scientiis*):

> Let this be laid down as a general rule: all divisions of knowledge should be understood and used in such a way that they mark and distinguish rather than cut and separate knowledge, in order always to avoid breaking the continuity among the various kinds of knowledge. The contrary approach has made individual disciplines barren, empty and straying, when they are not nourished, sustained and harmonized by a common source and fuel.[19]

---

18) *Ibid.,* 540.
19) *Ibid.,* 580.

Continuity of being (and matter) implies a continuity of knowledge, that is, *philosophia prima*. Bacon adds that he "unyokes" first philosophy from metaphysics: the former is "the common mother of sciences;" the latter "a part of natural philosophy."[20] Bacon describes *philosophia prima*, the ultimate root of knowledge, as "a repository of axioms" and "a hodgepodge (*farrago quaedam*), a confused mass (*massa incondita*) composed and put together from natural theology, logic and some parts of physics (the sections dealing with the principles and the soul)."[21] Axioms, in their being "common and promiscuous," are further evidence that one reality underlies unity of knowledge. Universal principles—such as: "Nature manifests itself most of all in the smallest things," "Everything changes, nothing perishes," "The death of one thing is postponed by being reduced to its principles," "What is capable of preserving a greater form is stronger in activity," "The power of an active principle is increased through the antiperistasis of the contrary principle"—find application in contexts as varied as physics, theology, moral philosophy and politics.[22]

Unity is therefore an original character of knowledge, for nature reflects itself in knowledge, and does not result from abstract representations projected onto and imposed upon reality (like lines converging into one focus). The axioms of *philosophia prima* do not point to "mere similarities (as they may appear to people who are not very perspicacious), but they are marks and signs (*vestigia et signacula*) imprinted on different matters and substrata." These *vestigia* and *signacula* are what Bacon calls "forms."[23] Even the part of *philosophia prima* that more specifically deals with the most general attributes of being (*conditiones adventitiae entium*, or *transcendentes*) demonstrates that philosophy is an investigation about natural reality, not according to the laws of language (*secundum naturae non sermonis leges*), nor in a supernatural sense.[24] By all

---

[20] *Ibid.*, 549.

[21] *Ibid.*, 540.

[22] *Ibid.*, 541-42, 550.

[23] *Ibid.*, 543. On the image of Pan's "horns" as the *ideae universales* or *summitates naturae* that, by touching heaven, connect metaphysics to natural theology, see *De sapientia veterum*, in *Works*, VI, 637, and n. 4. On Bacon's forms, see Antonio Pérez Ramos, *Francis Bacon's Idea of Science and the Maker's Knowledge Tradition* (Oxford, 1988).

[24] Bacon, *De augmentis scientiarum*, in *Works*, I, 544.

means, first philosophy deals with "nothing that is beyond nature, but with the most important part of nature" (*Certe ultra naturam nihil; sed ipsius naturae pars multo praestantissima*).[25] It considers such general attributes of being as "much" (*multum*) and "a little" (*paucum*), "like" (*simile*) and "unlike" (*diversum*), "possible" (*possibile*) and "impossible" (*impossibile*), the reasons why some natural beings can be found in nature in larger quantity than others, or why some creatures are more like animals and other more like plants.[26] *Philosophia prima* represents therefore the undifferentiated—"promiscuous" and "farraginous"—repository of notions (unlike *metaphysica*, which is the part of natural philosophy dealing with clearly defined and limited "forms").

Let us keep following Bacon a little more in his dichotomizing exercise. The inquiry into nature (*doctrina de natura*) is at the centre of Bacon's ontology. Nature represents the foundation of *philosophia prima*, which is the original core of knowledge from which the principal notions of natural philosophy emerge. Through the mediation of the "light of nature," nature is also the basis of the divine refractions studied by natural theology. Natural philosophy is then divided by Bacon into a theoretical part (*inquisitio causarum*) and an operative part (*productio effectuum*). The theoretical part of *philosophia naturalis* is further distinguished into *metaphysica* and *physica specialis*. *Metaphysica* is the most speculative part of physics. *Physica* is divided into three sections, one dealing with the most universal principles of nature (*de principiis rerum*), the second with the structure of the universe (*de fabrica universi*) and the third with nature studied in its aspects of scattered copiousness (*fusa et sparsa*) and individual diversity (*de varietate rerum*), which Bacon also describes as a "first gloss" to and a "paraphrasis" of the *interpretatio naturae*. Divisions do not end here, though, for he differentiates *physica sparsa* into concrete (*physica de concretis*) and abstract physics (*physica de abstractis*).[27]

---

25) *Ibid.*, 550.
26) *Ibid.*, 543-44. On the attribute of animal life in Bacon's philosophy, see Guido Giglioni, "The Uncomfortable *Biformitas* of Being: Bacon on the Animal Soul," in Cecilia Muratori, ed., *The Animal Soul and the Human Mind: Renaissance Debates* (Pisa and Rome, 2013), 192-207.
27) *Ibid.*, 551.

In all these divisions, Bacon acknowledges that he is using the term *metaphysica* in a sense that is "different from the received and ordinary one."[28] By all means, the way Bacon articulates the *doctrina de natura* into *physica* and *metaphysica* may remind us of Aristotle's division:

> Physics deal with the phenomena that are immersed in matter and are in motion (*mobilia*), metaphysics with the more abstract and stable ones (*constantia*). Also, in nature physics presupposes only existence, motion and natural necessity, while metaphysics adds mind and idea.[29]

Indeed, Bacon's account of the four causes looks even more Aristotelian: "Physics investigates the efficient cause and matter; metaphysics the form and the end."[30] In fact, the similarities are only apparent. For Bacon, *metaphysica*, and not *philosophia prima*, is a part of natural philosophy, while in Aristotle *metaphysica*, *philosophia prima* and *theologia* are internal articulations of the same discipline.[31]

Reason lifts over experience (while history and memory cling to it, and poesy and the imagination escape from it) and, by ascending through a series of increasingly more focused accounts of reality (*philosophia prima, physica sparsa, physica de concretis, physica de abstractis, metaphysica*), it leads from a *sylva* of countless "promiscuous" likenesses to a set of original forms in matter.[32] The metaphysical forms constitute the spelling-book of nature and our knowledge of them begins with spelling the alphabet of experience: *experientia literata*. Since there is no *solutio continuitatis* among the various degrees of knowledge, the alleged division between experimental and speculative philosophy in Bacon's work is an invention of modern interpreters, too concerned with issues of twentieth-century epistemology and loyalty to traditional atlases of philosophical legacies.

---

28) *Ibid.*, 550.

29) *Ibid.*

30) *Ibid.*

31) *Ibid.*, 551: "Cum vero omnis Physica sita sit in medio inter Historiam Naturalem et Metaphysicam, prior pars [i.e., *physica de concretis*] (si recte advertas) Historiae Naturali propior est; posterior [i.e. *physica de abstractis*] Metaphysicae."

32) See Guido Giglioni, "From the Woods of Experience to the Open Fields of Metaphysics: Bacon's Notion of *Silva*," forthcoming in *Renaissance Studies*.

3. Art of Discovery

In order to have a better understanding of the way in which Bacon describes the initial stages in human experience, we need to set *experientia literata* against the background of the principal divisions of knowledge. As already mentioned, Bacon's theory of knowledge presupposes a kind of psycho-physical parallelism between the human mind and nature. The foundational role that Bacon attributes to appetite—both the natural appetite of matter and the rational appetite of the human will—adds to the complexity of the parallelism.[33] Although two main disciplinary groups centred on logic and ethics are at the centre of the system of knowledge, Bacon maintains that the inquiry into the intellectual faculties (*doctrina circa intellectum*) is closely related to the inquiry into the will (*doctrina circa voluntatem*). Three are, in his opinion, the main reasons for this original relationship. The first is of an ontological order, and rests on the identity of the True with the Good.[34] The second concerns the theory of knowledge, and it is based on the link between the "purity of the illumination" and the "freedom of the will." The third reason, finally, has a theological foundation, and it refers to the fact that, after the Fall, human reason turned itself into a distorting ("menstruated") mirror as a result of the untameable nature of desire.[35] While logic deals with

---

[33] On the foundational role of material appetites in Bacon's philosophy, see Guido Giglioni, 'Francis Bacon', in Peter Anstey, ed., *The Oxford Handbook of British Philosophy in the Seventeenth Century* (Oxford, 2013), 41-72 (45-51); idem, *Francesco Bacone* (Rome, 2011), 59-95. On the role of the will in directing the process of knowledge, see Sorana Corneanu, *Regimens of the Mind: Boyle, Locke, and the Early Modern Cultura Animi Tradition* (Chicago and London, 2011), 14-45.

[34] Bacon, *De augmentis scientiarum*, in *Works*, I, 614: "Neque datur in universitate rerum tam intima sympathia, quam illa Veri et Boni."

[35] Bacon views any attempt to dissociate the alleged purity of knowledge from the contaminating effects of desire as a manifestation of intellectual prudery. See *De augmentis scientiarum*, in *Works*, I, 614: "Quo magis rubori fuerit viris doctis, si scientia sint tanquam angeli alati, cupiditatibus vero tanquam serpentes, qui humi reptant; circumgerentes animas instar speculi sane, sed menstruati." See also *ibid.*, 643: "sunt quidem Idola profundissimae mentis humanae fallaciae. Neque enim fallunt in particularibus, ut caeterae, judicio caliginem offundendo et tendiculas struendo; sed plane ex praedispositione mentis prava et perperam constituta, quae tanquam omnes intellectus anticipationes detorquet et inficit. Nam Mens Humana (corpore obducta et obfuscata) tantum abest ut speculo plano, aequali, et claro similis sit (quod rerum radios sincere

the operations of reason and the intellect, ethics focuses on the will, the appetite and the passions. The work of the imagination demonstrates that the two provinces of knowledge have a common origin (*in natalibus suis tanquam gemellae sunt*). Here the imagination, in its diplomatic capacity as a mediator between the two domains, is understood more as *phantasia* than *imaginatio*, that is to say, it conveys information (not always reliable) about reality rather than alter reality.[36]

> The senses deliver representations of all kinds (*idola omnigena*) to the imagination, and then reason judges them. In turn, before the decree is fulfilled, reason returns the representations back to the imagination after they have been selected and examined (*idola electa et probata*), for the imagination always precedes and stimulates the voluntary motion, so that the imagination is an instrument that is shared by both reason and the will.[37]

The imagination mediates, but it does not really produce knowledge by itself (*phantasia scientias fere non parit*). In this case, too, it is important to distinguish between *imaginatio* and *phantasia*. The principle of the imagination as *imaginatio* is nature, that of the imagination as *phantasia* is *poësis* (*poesy* in English), that is, the sheer power of fiction (*lusus ingenii* and not *scientia*).[38] Logic, in Bacon's opinion, has no need to rely on the lures of the imagination and the "meat" of the appetites, for the light of abstract knowledge is "dry" (*lumen siccum*).[39]

---

excipiat et reflectat), ut potius sit instar speculi alicujus incantati, pleni superstitionibus et spectris." For the image of the "menstruated" mirror, see Aristotle, *De insomniis*, II, 459b.

[36] Bacon, *De augmentis scientiarum*, in *Works*, I, 615: "Verum quidem est, quod Phantasia in utraque provincia, tam judiciali, quam ministeriali, legati cujusdam aut internuncii aut procuratoris reciproci vices gerit." On the difference between *imaginatio* and *phantasia* in Bacon, see Marta Fattori, "*Phantasia* nella classificazione baconiana delle scienze," in Fattori, ed., *Francis Bacon: Terminologia e fortuna nel XVII secolo* (Rome, 1984), 117-37; Guido Giglioni, "Fantasy Islands: *Utopia, The Tempest*, and *New Atlantis* as Places of Controlled Alienation," in Allison B. Kavey, ed., *World-Building and the Early Modern Imagination* (New York, 2010), 91-117. On imagination and *idola* in Bacon, see Sorana Corneanu and Koen Vermeir, "Idols of the Imagination: Francis Bacon on the Imagination and the Medicine of the Mind," *Perspectives on Science*, 20 (2012), 183-206.

[37] Bacon, *De augmentis scientiarum*, in *Works*, I, 615.

[38] *Ibid.*, 616.

[39] *Ibid.*: "Lumen siccum, optima anima," is how Bacon translates one of Heraclitus's fragments. See fr. 118, in Hermann Diels, ed., *Die Fragmente der Vorsokratiker. Griechisch*

Without apparently distancing himself too much from the classic partitions of the rhetorical tradition, Bacon articulates logic into four arts of reason (*artes rationales*), i.e., discovery, judgement, memory and delivery. The logic of discovery, which is the part of the system which concerns us the most in this discussion, refers to sciences and arts as well as to discourses and argumentations. Bacon acknowledges that more often than not in the history of humanity, great discoveries depended on luck and chance rather than knowledge of causes.[40] The example of medicine is clear evidence of this fact. Relying on Celsus' *De medicina*, Bacon points out that, in the history of medicine, discovery of remedies came first, later followed by discussions about their efficacy.[41] Indeed, the observation of the skilful behaviour of animals has often proved to be more productive than any study of logic. The ancients presented "animals, quadrupeds, birds, fish, snakes more than human beings as teachers of knowledge (*doctores scientiarum*)." Their relying on the inventive power of nature is witnessed by the many images of animals that adorn the temples of the Egyptians, a nation, Bacon reminds us, to which we owe the great majority of arts:

> regarding the discovery of arts, more than to dialectic, we are indebted to a wild goat for plasters, to a nightingale for musical melodies, to the ibis for cleansing the intestines, to the lid of a pot that burst asunder for artillery and, in a word, to chance or anything else.[42]

---

und Deutsch, 3 vols. (Berlin, 1922), I, 100. On the history of the interpretations concerning this fragment, see now Charles H. Kahn, *The Art and Thought of Heraclitus* (Cambridge, 2001), 245. The reference to the dry light of the intellect (*lumen siccum*), not drenched with the "oil" of the passions, recurs often in Bacon's works. See *Historia naturalis et experimentalis*, in *The* Instauratio Magna *Part II*: Historia Naturalis et Experimentalis: Historia Ventorum *and* Historia Vitae et Mortis, ed. Graham Rees with Maria Wakely (Oxford, 2007), OFB XII, 8; *Advancement of Learning*, ed. M. Kiernan (Oxford, 2000), OFB IV, 8; *Novum organum*, OFB XI, 87; *De sapientia veterum*, in *Works*, VI, 677.

[40] Bacon, *De augmentis scientiarum*, in *Works*, I, 617-18: "Quin et illi qui de primis rerum inventoribus aut scientiarum originibus verba fecerunt, casum potius quam artem celebrarunt."

[41] *Ibid.*, 617. Celsus's locus is also remembered in *Temporis partus masculus* (*Works*, III, 535) and *Redargutio philosophiarum* (*Works*, III, 578). See Celsus, *De medicina*, "Prooemium," 36.

[42] Bacon, *De augmentis scientiarum*, in *Works*, I, 618.

"Anything else," but not a method: Bacon has no hesitation in acknowledging that, at this stage of the discussion, he is focusing his attention on that "method of discovery" which also animals are capable of applying, that is, "an extremely acute attention (*attentissima sollicitudo*) addressed to one particular thing, and its continual exercise (*exercitatio*), attention and exercise that are imposed on these living beings by their need to survive (*sui conservandi necessitas*)."[43] Looking at the way animals organize themselves in nature, Bacon concludes that practice (*usus*) is a more powerful force than nature and art.[44] The examples of clever behaviour displayed by raven, bees and ants confirm that experience is the domain in which a skilful combination of *chance, cunning* and tendencies to *self-preservation* results in the best adaptations to reality and in the best inventions to improve such adaptations. The point is so important that Bacon waxes lyrical in describing the "ethereal dew of sciences" (*ros iste aethereus scientiarum*), that is, the distilled wisdom of nature which allows life to preserve itself while producing innovations of all sorts—and in doing so it fosters the critical shift from natural to artificial knowledge.[45] In *Redargutio philosophiarum*, Bacon points out how not a single experiment which did contribute to the betterment of human condition has been drawn from philosophical speculations, "laboured and polished in the course of so many years," so much so that one might say that "the animals' instincts have brought about more discoveries than the words of learned men."[46]

To confirm his view that the models of induction devised by dialecticians and rhetoricians have almost no impact on the way in which we organize and improve our knowledge, Bacon uses a number of significant terms drawn from Cicero, Virgil and Persius, such as *sollicitudo, sollertia, sagacitas, exercitatio, industria, usus* and *labor*. It is certainly not by chance (or for decorative reasons) that in these pages of *De augmentis scientiarum* Bacon refers more than once to Virgil's *Georgics*. The natural inductions on which both animals and farmers rely are much more pro-

---

[43] *Ibid.*, 618-19.
[44] The reference is to Cicero, *Pro Balbo*, 20.
[45] Bacon, *De augmentis scientiarum*, in *Works*, I, 619-20. Compare the *ros aethereus* of the sciences with the *aura quaedam vitalis* whereby the mechanical arts grow and are perfected by the day: *Cogitata et visa*, in *Works*, III, 616.
[46] Bacon, *Redargutio philosophiarum*, in *Works*, III, 578.

ductive than the inductive procedures described in textbooks of logic. In natural inductions, "sciences are drawn from particular instances, partly natural, partly artificial, like flowers, of both meadow and garden." By contrast, in the case of textbook inductions, significantly characterized by Bacon as crude (*pinguis*) and coarse (*crassa*), "the simple enumeration of particulars" can only lead to the domain of "probable conjecture."[47] The reason why the so-called inductions *per enumerationem simplicem* do not result in any real discovery—and instead they obstruct rather than promote the progress of knowledge—is that no confirmation of sense data can ever produce new results by itself; on the contrary, this validation, comforting as it may be, reinforces prejudices and drives one to go along the same route over and over again (*repetitio infinita*). Knowledge grows and thrives through questions—and Bacon has no qualms about acknowledging that we can master questions more than things (*domini enim quaestionum sumus, rerum non item*)—but questions emerge from the human mind only when this is confronted (painfully so, in most cases) by negative responses, disenchanting experiences, refutations and surprises.[48]

In *Redargutio philosophiarum*, Bacon compares the useless exercises of logic to the dinner of the "host from Chalcis" mentioned by the Roman historian Livy. Having been asked about the provenance of the sumptuous dishes of game served up on the table, the witty host answered that it was simply pork dressed with all sorts of spices and seasonings. Likewise, Bacon continues, "all this wealth of knowledge is only a portion of the philosophy of the Greeks, which did not feed upon pastures and woods in nature, but upon schools and cells, like a domestic animal reared in a farm."[49] However, Bacon has no intention of transforming knowledge into a completely natural process, for in this case experience would never progress from the stage of illiteracy (*experientia illiterata*)

---

[47] Bacon, *De augmentis scientiarum*, in *Works*, I, 620.

[48] *Ibid.*, 639: "Domini enim quaestionum sumus, rerum non item." See also *Redargutio philosophiarum*, in *Works*, III, 560. On Bacon's effort to find ways of controlling deeply-ingrained tendencies to delusion and self-delusion in human nature, see Guido Giglioni, "Philosophy according to Tacitus: Francis Bacon and the Inquiry into the Limits of Human Self-Delusion," *Perspectives on Science*, 20 (2012), 159-82.

[49] Bacon, *Redargutio philosophiarum*, in *Works*, III, 560-61. Cf. Livy, *Historiae*, XXXV, 49.

to technological expertise. To refer to another metaphor used by Bacon, in the wild territories of experience (*saltus apertus*) we proceed from one particular to another, from one experiment to another; in the gardens of experience (*vivaria*), knowledge is being organized in topics and repositories of places and subjects. The former are as it were *natural particulars*, the latter *artificial particulars*. Bacon assigns great value to specific commonplaces, understood as collections of "places of investigation and discovery, specific for particular subjects and kinds of knowledge." These "places" are described as "mixtures of logic and matter," where "matter" means the specific content of particular sciences."[50]

> It is obvious that he who thinks that the art of discovering knowledge can be devised and presented as complete from the beginning (and is to be applied and practised as such) is a fatuous and narrow-minded person. Human beings should know that *the arts of discovery grow in solidity and truth and that they grow together with what has been discovered up to that point.*[51]

Inventio is therefore a cognitive process in which categories and objects adjust to each other in the very process of knowledge. In this, Bacon advocates a notion of "impure" reason. Just as there cannot be real *philosophia* without *historia*, in the same way, the logic of discovery cannot be separated from the object that one intends to know. It is like undertaking a journey and becoming gradually accustomed to the distance to cover and the final destination: cognitive strategies and objects of knowledge calibrate their targets and scopes by constantly measuring each other.[52]

---

[50] Bacon, *De augmentis scientiarum*, in *Works*, I, 635: "Illi autem mixturae quaedam sunt, ex logica et materia ipsa propria singularum scientiarum."

[51] *Ibid.*, 636. And he goes on: "adeo ut cum quis primum ad perscrutationem scientiae alicujus accesserit, possit habere praecepta inventivae nonnulla utilia; postquam autem ampliores in ipsa scientia progressus fecerit, possit etiam et debeat nova inventionis praecepta excogitare, quae ad ulteriora eum foelicius deducant." Cf. *ibid.*, 639: "Illum interim, quod monere occoepimus, iterum monemus; nempe ut homines debeant topicas particulares suas alternare, ita ut post majores progressus aliquos in inquisitione factos aliam et subinde aliam instituant topicam, si modo scientiarum fastigia conscendere cupiant."

[52] *Ibid.*, 636. On the relationship between *philosophia* and *historia* in Bacon and his view of "impure" reason, see Guido Giglioni, "*Historia* and *Materia*: The Philosophical

The "impurity" of Baconian reason becomes even more evident when we examine the passage from nature to skill, for the shift from natural ability to methodical knowledge occurs through language. The transition is particularly delicate in Bacon's philosophy, as the alphabet of natural experience in its vital immediacy needs to be translated into the artificial code of human knowledge. Language can easily upset the balance of logic and matter in the "mixture" underlying topical places. In those disciplines that Bacon calls "popular" (*scientiae populares*), "such as moral philosophy, politics, jurisprudence and the like" (even in theology, every time God condescends to the minds of human beings), we can proceed through syllogisms, for in this case the exchange of information depends on notions that are linguistically structured. However, in our knowledge of natural reality (*in physicis*), where nature needs to be confronted with concrete and immediate results, and does not behave like an "adversary" that we have to win over through arguments, "truth slips from one's hands, for nature's operations are subtler than words."[53] Syllogisms are made up of propositions, these of words, and words are tokens of concepts (*tesserae notionum*). Therefore, "if concepts (which are the soul of words) are abstracted from things in an incorrect and inconstant way, the whole edifice of knowledge crumbles down (*tota fabrica corruit*)."[54] Moreover, "no laborious analysis of the consequences of the arguments or the truth of the propositions will ever restore the thing (*res*) in its entirety, since, as physicians say, the fault takes shape in the 'first digestion' (*prima digestione*), and it is not corrected by the following functions."[55]

The transition from natural to artificial experience (or to use again Bacon's images and examples, the shift from "meadow" to "garden," from goats to doctors and from birds to musicians) is of the utmost importance for Bacon, for the whole point in establishing a process of cognitive literacy (*experientia literata*) is precisely to show how we acquire the skill to interpret nature (*novum organum*) and proceed to the larger pro-

Implications of Francis Bacon's Natural History," *Early Science and Medicine*, 17 (2012), 62-86.

[53] Bacon, *De augmentis scientiarum*, in *Works*, I, 621.
[54] *Ibid.*, 621.
[55] *Ibid.*

gramme of reforming and transforming reality (*instauratio*).[56] Language has a key role in transforming natural into artificial information and organizing our knowledge of nature into categories (commonplaces as *mixturae ex logica et materia*). There is an original language of nature, which Bacon calls the alphabet of nature and which consists of the primordial constituents of reality (motions and appetites), and there is the human language understood as an artificial construction which, as one of the "idols of the market-place" (*idola fori*), may contribute to alienate the human mind from reality. The idea of comparing a limited number of original appetites in matter to the letters of the alphabet is a recurrent motif in Bacon's writings.[57] In the work *Abecedarium novum naturae* ("A new spelling-book of nature"), composed in all likelihood during the year 1622, the comparison is examined at length and the various elements belonging to the analogy between experience and literacy are discussed: the alphabet, the spelling-book and the book of nature. The image of the alphabet brings epistemological and ontological issues together. The main distinction is between the original characters of nature, i.e., the primal appetites of matter, and the spelling-book of nature, i.e., the method through which we learn the language of matter as if we were children. "I have composed and published this spelling-book," says Bacon at the beginning of the tract, "nothing special or official, but I had in mind what children do (*imitatio puerilis*), which nevertheless is absolutely to the point, for it is aimed at the kingdom of man, which consists in knowledge, in the same way as in the heavenly kingdom entry is not allowed unless one is like a child." Bacon then goes on and places the phase of cognitive literacy well within the broader philosophical project of mending our broken ties with nature (*instauratio*): "this spelling-book belongs to the fourth part of the Instauration, which is the ladder or machine of the intellect."[58] The spelling-book of nature is concerned only with the original, irreducible forms of matter, the forms that constitute all beings

---

[56] On the relationship between nature and art, see Sophie Weeks, "Francis Bacon and the Art-Nature Distinction," *Ambix*, 54 (2007), 117-45.

[57] Bacon, *Valerius Terminus*, in *Works*, III, 243; *Cogitationes de natura rerum*, in *Works*, III, 22; *Advancement of Learning*, OFB IV, 84.

[58] Francis Bacon, *Abecedarium novum naturae*, in *The* Instauratio Magna: *Last Writings*, ed. Graham Rees (Oxford, 2000), OFB XIII, 172. On the *Abecedarium*, see Graham Rees, "Introduction," in *ibid.*, xxxvi-xlviii.

of nature. Such a spelling-book, says Bacon, "does not analyse the matter down to the most specific species (*infimae species*)," for "the letters of the alphabet should not be confused with syllables and words."[59] By mastering the original letters of nature's language and by undertaking—more or less tentatively—the first experimental exercises, the human mind becomes better equipped for the more complicated task of interpreting nature. This is the way Bacon presents the matter in *Cogitationes de natura rerum* ("Thoughts on nature"):

> To be sure, just as the words and names of all languages, in their vast variety, consist of few simple letters (*paucae literae simplices*), in the same way, all actions and powers of things result from few natures and causes of simple motions. It is a shame that human beings have put so much effort in studying the tinkling of their own voices (*propriae vocis tintinnabula*), while they remain in this state of illiteracy with respect to the voice of nature (*ad naturae autem vocem tam illiteratos esse*); and, as if they were at the dawn of time (before the discovery of writing), they only recognize compounded sounds and words, but do not distinguish elements and letters.[60]

If therefore errors resulting from hasty apprehensions or dogmatic anticipations accrue in words and languages, it is important to intervene at the level of the "first digestion" or go back to the initial steps in knowledge when we learnt to spell the language of nature, and to see to it that sense perceptions are not falsified by inadequate notions and words. In the domain of sense knowledge, to capitulate to a kind of scepticism that mistrusts the power of the senses represents for Bacon the principal error of the philosophical tradition, and this sceptical attitude has become even more detrimental once it associated itself with the nonchalant attitude towards reality that is characteristic of rhetoricians. Being more interested in displaying their argumentative abilities and indifferent about the subjects they happen to defend, they have perpetuated an incantatory use of language and words. In Bacon's opinion, Cicero is a typical representative of this mixture of rhetorical frivolity and bland scepticism.[61]

The most serious mistake of all, however, has been that of "calumniate" sense perceptions. By doing so, sceptics and rhetoricians have destroyed

---

[59] Bacon, *Abecedarium novum naturae*, OFB XIII, 90.

[60] Bacon, *Cogitationes de natura rerum*, in *Works*, III, 22.

[61] Bacon, *De augmentis scientiarum*, in *Works*, I, 622.

knowledge from its foundations (*unde Scientias radicitus evellebant*).[62]
Bacon's main concern is that, by challenging the reliability of the senses,
sceptics deny the possibility that natural skill, with its array of adaptive
abilities, may evolve to cognitive functions of a higher level. Demonstrating the reliability of experimental knowledge is the first step to answer
the objections coming from the sceptics and to move from natural to
artificial experience:

> Although the senses often deceive or desert human beings, nevertheless, they can
> meet the requirements of knowledge when they are assisted by assiduous activity;
> and this may happen not so much by applying instruments (although they contrib-
> ute to this end), as through that kind of experiments which are able to produce
> objects that are subtler (*objecta subtiliora*) than the ones that can be grasped by
> the senses.[63]

The cause responsible of altering the natural "digestion" of knowledge
should not be sought for in the senses, but in the mind, which—also as
a result of the Fall—refrains from submitting itself to the reality of things
(what Bacon calls the mind's "contumacy," such that it "refuses to comply
with reality"). This does not mean that the intellect should be excluded
from participating in the enterprise of knowledge. It needs "helps"
(*auxilia*) that prevent it from drifting away from reality and a "prepara-
tion" (*praeparatio*) that predisposes it to the work of knowledge:

> No one has a hand so steady (nor can he acquire it through exercise) that he can
> draw a straight line or a perfect circle freehand; by contrast, this can be easily done
> by using a ruler or a compass. This is the real target (*res ipsa*) towards which we are
> striving with all our forces, i.e., that the mind, through discipline, may become a
> match to reality (*ut scilicet mens per artem fiat rebus par*).[64]

That the mind may realign itself to reality, so that it will be like it was at
the beginning of the creation, is the goal of the *ars* of "clue and direction."
The art of finding clues, Bacon continues, consists of two parts, for the
indicium can be obtained by proceeding from one experiment to

---

[62] *Ibid.*

[63] *Ibid.*

[64] *Ibid.* On the question of the aids for the process of knowledge, see Stewart, "*Res,
veluti per Machinas, Conficiatur.*"

another (*ab experimentis ad experimenta*), or by drawing axioms from experiments, and then new experiments from the axioms that have been obtained in this way. Bacon calls the first part of this art cognitive literacy (*experientia literata*), that is, the process through which we learn the first rudiments of knowledge, the second part, the "interpretation of nature, or new organ" (*interpretatio naturae, sive novum organum*), through which we apply our reading skills to the complex task of explaining the structures of reality.[65]

4. *Experientia literata*

When dwelling on the question of how human beings grasp the first rudiments of experience, Bacon draws an analogy between the process through which children learn to spell and read and the one through which human beings make experience of the surrounding reality. Although grownups consider it to be a demeaning experience to go back to the "the first elements of inductions" and to read and revise "like children," Bacon suggests that in order to build the edifice of knowledge on solid foundations one should do the same with the language of nature: we spell words by telling their letters, we know bodies by identifying their constituent appetites.[66] Bacon makes clear that the process of gaining experiential literacy is not a form of philosophical knowledge, but a kind of natural acumen (*sagacitas quaedam*). In emblematic terms, as often is the case with Bacon, this experience is also called "Pan's hunt" (*venatio Panis*):[67]

> there are three ways in which one can proceed in this manner: by groping around in the dark (*cum palpat ipse in tenebris*); by being led by hand by someone who is

---

[65] Bacon, *De augmentis scientiarum*, in *Works*, I, 623.

[66] *Ibid.*, 620-21: "Quemadmodum enim in Divina Veritate percipienda aegre quis in animum inducat ut fiat tanquam parvulus; ita in humana perdiscenda, provectos utique, puerorum more, prima inductionum elementa adhuc legere et retractare, res humilis existimatur et quasi contemnenda." See also *Historia naturalis et experimentalis*, in OFB XII, 10. Cf. Mt 18,3: "nisi conversi fueritis et efficiamini sicut parvuli non intrabitis in regnum caelorum."

[67] Bacon, *De augmentis scientiarum*, in *Works*, I, 623. See *De sapientia veterum*, in *Works*, VI, 635-41: "Potestates ei [Pani] et munera hujusmodi attribuuntur, ut sit deus venatorum, etiam pastorum, et in universum ruricolarum."

also not seeing very well (*cum alterius manu ducatur, ipse parum videns*); or, finally, by following traces using a light (*cum vestigia lumine adhibito regat*). In the same way, one may try experiments of all kinds without following any pattern or method, and this is a mere feeling by touch (*mera palpatio*). One may use some direction and order in experimenting, and it is like being led by hand: this is what we mean by *experientia literata*. For the light, which is the third option, is needed in the case of the interpretation of nature, also known as "new organ."[68]

Between the stage in which we are barely capable of making sense of an overwhelming mass of disjointed and ambiguous stimuli, data, hints and clues (*experientia illiterata*), and that in which we finally master the art of reading the text of nature both fluently and critically (*interpretatio naturae*), the human mind undergoes a process through which it learns to put its knowledge to the test. In making experience of things, the mind is not overpowered by them; at the same time, though, it is not ready yet to disclose their meaning. It spells out the "characters" and "letters" of experience, and tentatively read the book of nature, but it does not grasp yet the larger structures of meaning that constitute the building blocks underlying the human understanding of the world. In other words, the *experientia literata* cannot break the circle—sometimes virtuous, sometimes vicious—of experiments and find a way out of the woods of experience. As such, it deals with a whole array of experimental strategies (*modi experimentandi*), that is, with the many ways in which we organize our experience in order to outline the primary patterns of knowledge.[69]

Bacon divides the experimental forms of knowledge into eight types, which represent a number of elementary cognitive procedures through which the mind remains as flexible as possible towards experience. Experiments can be organized through "variation" (*variatio*), "protraction" (*productio*), "transfer" (*translatio*), "inversion" (*inversio*), "constraint," (*compulsio*), "application" (*applicatio*), "coupling" (*copulatio*) and "by chance" (*sortes*). As far as the mode of "variation" is concerned, this can be applied every time one observes how specific natural phenomena develop by varying the experimental setting through a number of variables: matter (for instance, when one can produce different kinds of paper using different materials, or when new varieties of plants and flowers

---

[68] Bacon, *De augmentis scientiarum*, in *Works*, I, 623.
[69] See *Novum organum*, OFB XI, 160.

are created by changing the type of graft); the efficient principle (examples are: increasing the intensity of radiations coming from the moon by using lenses that are different from the ones employed with solar rays, or arranging experiments which demonstrate that magnetism can also be caused by heat); and quantity (for example, when we observe the differences created by increasing or diminishing the quantity of a specific substance or the intensity of a force). "Protraction" of experiments occurs through "repetition," every time we replicate an experiment (*cum experimentum iteratur*) so that we can establish the limits of a specific phenomenon, or when we resort to "extension" (*cum ad subtilius quiddam urgetur*), so that we can observe a phenomenon reduced to its minimal conditions. Experimental "transfer" happens in three ways: from nature or chance to art (i.e., artificial imitation of natural phenomena); from one kind of art or practice to another; or from one part to another within the confines of the same art. We have "inversion" of experiments when we plan to study the different effects that result from organizing opposite and complementary settings, as in the case of experiments concerning heat and cold. Experimental "constraints" happen every time an experiment "is pressed and protracted until one specific force is annihilated or released," that is, when we set up such experimental conditions that one phenomenon is brought to the limits of its specific nature (e.g., the limits of attraction for a loadstone, or the limits of magnification for a specific lens). "Application" of experiments presupposes the ability to adapt the results that are valid for a specific experiment to a different experimental setting (*ingeniosa traductio*) so that we may gather new valuable information. "Men should keep their eyes wide open," Bacon points out at this point, "and turn their attention to the nature of things, on the one hand, and to their uses, on the other."[70] Experiments belong to the heading "coupling" when they refer to all those cases in which the effects of a particular experiment are enhanced when they are combined with those of another one.

Despite being the most elusive of all, the last experiential modality—that "by chance"—is perhaps the most important one given the central role that Bacon assigned to chance in shaping *experientia literata*:

---

[70] Bacon, *De augmentis scientiarum*, in *Works*, I, 631.

This way of experimenting is wholly irrational and, as it were, insane (*furiosus*). It takes place when you realize that you can try something not because you have been led to do so by reason or by some other experiment, but simply because that attempt has never been done before.[71]

Bacon maintains that a fundamental cognitive principle lies in this kind of *experientia literata*, i.e., the idea that no possibility should be left untried, that no stone should be left unturned—*omnem lapidem in natura moveas*. The fact is, Bacon continues, that "the great works of nature (*magnalia naturae*) can be found outside the common routes and known tracks, so that sometimes the very absurd character of the thing may be of help."[72]

To the extent that it contributes to refute a hypothesis or to reveal how disappointing the promises of one particular theory may be, chance has the power to shed new light on old assumptions or disclose paths unknown up to that point. Closely connected to the question of random discoveries is the one of failure, understood either as an unsuccessful experiment or an unexpected result. It is precisely the inevitable limitations of the *experientia literata* that leads to overcome the level of experience for experience's sake, no matter how successful and productive this may be, and to open up new possibilities for human knowledge. To keep using the metaphorical armoury associated with Bacon's *experientia literata*, pure spelling without reading or simple reading without interpreting does not lead to discover the meaning of the book of nature. It is clear why light-bearing experiments (*experimenta lucifera*) are more important than fruit-bearing ones (*experimenta fructifera*).[73] More than practical results, it is the growth in awareness that triggers the interpretative activity and expands the range of inductive reasoning.

---

[71] *Ibid.*, 632. See *Cogitata et visa*, in *Works*, III, 614: "Casum nimirum proculdubio multis inventis principium dedisse, sumpta ex natura rerum occasione." The difference between *casus* and *ars* is that the former occurs at the last minute, in a sporadic and scattered way, while the latter proceeds by drawing up the "troops" of knowledge in an orderly and economic fashion: "Casum enim operari raro, et sero, et sparsim; Artem contra constanter, et compendio, et turmatim" (*ibid.*).

[72] Bacon, *De augmentis scientiarum*, in *Works*, I, 632. See *Cogitata et visa*, in *Works*, III, 615: "eandem et eorum quae in sinu naturae adhuc recondita sunt magna ex parte rationem esse, ut hominum imaginationes et commentationes fugiant et fallant."

[73] Bacon, *De augmentis scientiarum*, in *Works*, I, 632-33.

The interplay of experience, chance and cognitive drive finds a magnificent emblematic representation in Bacon's *De sapientia veterum* ("The Wisdom of the Ancients"). Pan, whose hunt is described as *experientia literata* in *De augmentis scientiarum*, is an emblem of both nature (*Universitas Rerum sive Natura*) and experience (*experientia sagax et rerum mundi notitia universalis*).[74]

> Pan's office could not be represented and displayed in more lively terms than as being the god of hunters, for every natural action—and therefore motion and process—is nothing but hunting. Arts and sciences hunt for their works, human assemblies hunt for their deliberations, and all things of nature (*res naturales omnes*) hunt either for their food as their prey, or for their pleasure as a source of relief. And they do this in ways that are expert and sagacious.[75]

There is an important element of randomness in Pan's activities. When Ceres decided to hide herself because angry at the rape of her daughter Proserpina, "for some happy chance, only Pan happened to find and reveal Ceres while he was hunting." Bacon stresses the fact that Ceres was found by Pan "while hunting" (*inter venandum; inter venationem*): "the discovery of things useful for life and civilization," like agriculture (*seges*), is not expected from "abstract philosophies" (i.e., higher goods), all intent to reach this end (*licet totis viribus in illud ipsum incumbant*), but from the haphazard and yet sagacious experience of Pan, who "by chance" runs into "findings of this kind."[76]

As I argued at the beginning of this article, there is no way that, when dealing with Bacon's philosophy, we can separate the level of discussion concerning knowledge from the one concerning nature, and imagine epistemological concerns dissociated from ontological commitments, or experimental practices divorced from speculative interests. Pan symbolizes both nature and knowledge; better, it is nature's own chase towards self-knowledge and form. And no doubt, at the end of his life, in the intricate pathways of the *Sylva Sylvarum*, Bacon was Pan chasing his own Ceres.

---

74) Bacon, *De sapientia veterum*, in *Works*, VI, 635-36. See also *De augmentis scientiarm*, in *Works*, I, 521-30.

75) Bacon, *De sapientia veterum*, in *Works*, VI, 638.

76) *Ibid.*, 640.

5. Conclusion

To recapitulate, the *modi experimentandi* outlined by Bacon in the art of clue and direction show that a number of skills are integral to the constitution of one's experiential literacy: natural shrewdness, keenness of scent (*odoratio venatica*), the ability to recognize significant clues, the capability of adapting already acquired information to contexts of different nature, an elementary power of sentient discernment, still entangled in countless sensible clues, and a determination to proceed by trial and error even when there seems to be no reason for doing so.[77] Transfer of experiments from one disciplinary domain to another is a way of maximising the productivity of chance in the absence of a clear interpretative theory. The ability to spot connections among experiments requires acumen. "Nature is the mirror of art," Bacon argues, and for those people who do not know the forms and causes of matter, the mirror of nature provides reflections that can be usefully put to fruition in different disciplines. The sudden and unforeseen explosion of a distillatory apparatus, for instance, is likely to have led the alchemist monk to think of a possible analogy between the explosion in his kitchen and the thunder and lightning in the sky:

> nothing can contribute to a shower, so to speak, of useful and new inventions, falling as it were from the sky, more than when experiments from various mechanical arts are brought to the attention of someone or a group of people who can sharpen their minds by discussing the matter together. In this way, through what we have called "transfer of experiments," disciplines (*artes*) can be stimulated and kindled as through a concentration of rays, for, although the rational path that passes through the Organ promises far greater results, nevertheless, this kind of sagacity through experiential literacy (*experientia literata*) sometimes hurls and scatters a large amount of inventions that are within reach of mankind (as the gifts that ancient emperors used to throw among their people).[78]

A pyrotechnic explosion of new discoveries: this is the way Bacon describes the effects of *experientia literata*. Paradoxically, loose experiment-

---

[77] Bacon, *De augmentis scientiarum*, in *Works*, I, 626: "Judicium igitur in hac re adhibendum"; *ibid.*, 633: *experientia literata* is "*Sagacitas* potius ... et odoratio quaedam venatica, quam *Scientia*."

[78] Bacon, *De augmentis scientiarum*, in *Works*, I, 628-29.

ing has a remarkable advantage when compared to a clearly defined set of methodological rules (the "Organ"): the very absence of norms. The possibility of trying all the available options, even the most improbable and arbitrary ones, expands immeasurably the field of what can be experimented and the freedom of the experimenter. In doing so, *experientia literata* re-enacts the situation of productive dispersal represented by the original *sylva* of experience.

But it is precisely in the darkness of the wood that knowledge must start. In one of the *Meditationes sacrae* ("Sacred meditations"), Bacon connects sagacity to the need of "medicining" one's mind (*inutiliter adhibetur medicina non pertentato vulnere*) and to the importance of striking a balance between the self-sufficiency of nature (*columbina innocentia*) and the indefatigably probing tendency of the mind (*serpentina prudentia*):[79]

> he who aspires to a kind of goodness which is not withdrawn and individual, but diffusive (*seminalis*) and productive (*genitiva*), such that other people may be attracted to it, must by all means become acquainted with what the Evangelist calls the depths of Satan (*profunda Satanae*), so that he can speak with authority and true endorsement. Hence the saying: "Prove all things; hold fast to that which is good," which suggests a judicious choice out of a universal examination.[80]

As we have just seen, one of the distinguishing features of *experientia literata* lies in its being *plane irrationalis et quasi furiosa*. No doubt, nothing can be more irrational and mad than delving into the depths of Satan. And yet even in this case Bacon cannot help seeing the positive and productive aspect of human experience—*et sol ingreditur latrinas, nec inquinatur*.[81]

---

[79] Bacon, *Meditationes sacrae*, in *Works*, VII, 234: "Judicio hominis depravato et corrupto, omnis quae adhibetur eruditio et persuasio irrita est et despectui, quae non ducit exordium a detectione et repraesentatione malae complexionis animi sanandi; quemadmodum inutiliter adhibeatur medicina non pertentato vulnere." *Pertentare vulnus* refers here to the surgeon's action of examining the nature of a wound by touching and feeling the affected area. Bacon expands on the importance of "medicining" one's mind before pursuing knowledge of reality in *Advancement of Learning*, OFB IV, 149.

[80] Bacon, *Meditationes sacrae*, in *Works*, VII, 234-35. See Apc 2, 24: "altitudines Satanae"; 1 Ts 5,21: "Omnia autem probate, quod bonum est tenete."

[81] Bacon, *Meditationes sacrae*, in *Works*, VII, 235.

Of Snails and Horsetails:
Anatomical Empiricism in the Early Modern Period

Domenico Bertoloni Meli
Indiana University, Bloomington*

Abstract

The problem of generalization was a vexing one in anatomical investigations: when was it legitimate to generalize from one individual observed or dissected at a given time to the same individual at different times, or to individuals of the same species, or even to individuals from different species altogether? Views on these matters varied widely from the Renaissance to the Enlightenment and guided different research programs based on opposite assumptions. A growing basis of empirical results made anatomists aware of the dangers of hasty generalizations. The problem of reproduction in animals and plants led to especially startling findings that shattered naïve assumptions about the uniformity of nature. Yet, from a multitude of seemingly unpredictable results, new, equally unpredictable patterns and analogies emerged, leading to the discovery of sexual reproduction in plants, for example. Snails and horsetails proved especially challenging in this context.

Keywords

empiricism, comparative anatomy, sexual reproduction, generalization

Introduction

The empirical medical tradition has often been associated with a school in antiquity questioning the search for causes and anatomical knowledge; by contrast, the dogmatist or rationalist school would emphasize causes and anatomical knowledge. Different incarnations of these views were very much alive in the early modern period, with those like Thomas Sydenham, for example, questioning the role of anatomy and

---
* Indiana University, Bloomington, 1011 E. Third St., Goodbody Hall 130, Bloomington, IN 47405, USA (dbmeli@indiana.edu).

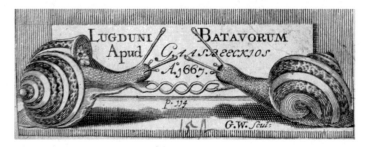

Figure 1: This figure, from the title page of Jan Swammerdam, *De respiratione* (Leiden, 1667) is reproduced by courtesy of the Lilly Library, Indiana University, Bloomington

the search for causes, whereas others were making precisely of these aspects the focus of their investigations. In a peculiar way, however, followers of the empirical tradition relied on generalization, in the sense that a remedy that was proved effective on one occasion was applied again and again by imitation until it was considered part of their art. By contrast, the rationalist school relied on the key features of each individual case with regard to both the temperament of each patient and the climate and situation of where patients lived. Thus, at least if we are to follow what Galen tells us in *De sectis*, the empirical tradition relies on the general whereas the rationalist relies on the particular.[1]

In this brief essay, I address the issue of medical empiricism from a different perspective, focusing not primarily on therapy but rather on anatomy and more specifically on the problem of generalization of knowledge and the tension between the uniformity and diversity of nature. In order to come to grips with this issue, I wish to consider three levels of diversity: diversity among species; diversity among organisms within a species; and diversity within an individual organism, with regard to age, for example. These three levels provide a structure for my essay.

The two perspectives that I have outlined—one based primarily on therapies and the other on anatomy—are not entirely unrelated, because the anatomical study of diversity within an organism, or among organisms within the same species, for example, have profound medical and therapeutic implications; moreover, in the early modern period and pos-

---

[1] Galen, *De sectis*, in *Three Treatises on the Nature of Science*, transl. Richard Walzer and Michael Frede (Indianapolis, 1985), esp. 4-5.

sibly even more so today, different animal species were used for physiological and medical investigations, with differences among species proving of crucial significance: as we are constantly reminded in media reports, testing a new chemical on mice is one thing, testing it on humans another.

The time from the Renaissance to the Enlightenment witnessed a growing tension between views on uniformity and diversity in nature. While some believed that nature operates according to an ever constant necessity and that every variation observed could be seen as a subtle modulation on a fundamentally homogeneous pattern, others argued that nature's uniformity is a myth and that only painstaking empirical investigations can reveal her mysteries: snails and horsetails took an important role in those debates. The Bolognese anatomist Marcello Malpighi was an especially prominent voice in the camp defending uniformity. In his works we read many statements such as the following: "Since nature's constant way of operating is one and the same, in macroscopic and microscopic parts" (1666); "We see nature proceeding with one simple method" (1689); "Nature, that operates with an ever uniform necessity" (1697).[2] Yet, despite his own methodological predicaments, Malpighi's own findings often led to results that he and his contemporaries alike found startling. My preliminary reflections in this essay seek to begin unraveling some issues arising from this tension.

1. Diversity among Species

Animals and plants, in short, all living organisms, present striking diversities at many levels, making generalizations from species to species problematic. Presumably humans have always been aware of this diversity, though the specific form of this awareness and the nature of the research carried out to investigate it changed with time, occasionally in dramatic fashion. The exact meaning of the expression "anatomia comparata" changed over time: the expression was used and possibly coined by Francis Bacon in *The Advancement of Learning* to mean a comparison

---

[2] Marcello Malpighi, *Correspondence*, ed. Howard B. Adelmann, 5 vols. (Ithaca, 1975), 2: 802n3.

among the individuals of a species, not different species, as we do today and as I will do in this essay.[3]

In the early 1520s, the surgeon and anatomist Jacopo Berengario da Carpi highlighted the need to dissect animals of different species, age, sex, both pregnant and not pregnant, living and dead, thus indicating his methodological and epistemological awareness about several themes addressed in this essay. It was Berengario who questioned the existence of the *rete mirabile* in humans well before Andreas Vesalius: the *rete mirabile* is a network of arteries found at the base of the brain in sheep and other ungulates, as well as in other animals, though not in humans. Vesalius made of the realization that Galen had not dissected humans a key tenet of his monumental work, the *De humani corporis fabrica*: it was precisely because humans differ from animals and because Galen had not dissected humans and had been deceived by his monkeys and other animals that Vesalius's *Fabrica* was such a key text. In the late Renaissance the growing interest in comparative anatomy in the works by the Padua anatomist Hieronymus Fabricius, William Harvey, and his correspondent, the distinguished Neapolitan physician and surgeon Marco Aurelio Severino, led to a number of investigations on all sorts of animals from insects and shrimps to deer. Karin Ekholm, for example, has recently shown that Fabricius identified a huge variability in the placentas of different animals, which he grouped in four different types; placentas can differ so much from species to species that they could hardly be identified purely on structural grounds. The growing awareness of diversity increased in the seventeenth century as well, fueled by European colonial enterprises, with the increasing number of rare and exotic animals filling menageries of princes and kings, from elephants to beavers and camels, as Anita Guerrini has recently shown.[4]

---

[3]   Francis J. Cole, *A History of Comparative Anatomy* (London, 1944) 10. Francis Bacon, *Of Proficience and Advancement of Learning* (London, 1605), book 2, section X.5.

[4]   Andreas Vesalius, *De humani corporis fabrica* (Basel, 1543), dedication to Charles V. Katharine Park, *Secrets of Women. Gender, Generation, and the Origins of Human Dissection* (Brooklyn, NY, 2006) 168. Cole, *Comparative Anatomy*, sections xi-xiv. Karin J. Ekholm, "Fabricius's and Harvey's Representations of Animal Generation," *Annals of Science*, 67 (2010), 329-52. Anita Guerrini, "The King's Animals and the King's Books: The Illustrations for the Paris Academy's *Histoire des animaux*," *Annals of Science*, 67 (2010), 383-404. Vivian Nutton, "Introduction" to *On the Fabric of the Human Body*, transl. Daniel Garrison and Malcolm Hast, at http://vesalius.northwestern.edu/flash.html

"Anatomia comparata" was exceedingly challenging even for seasoned investigators. A feel for the dangers of this field and the difficulty in identifying organs and body parts in unusual animals can be gained from this comment by the comparative anatomist and historian Francis J. Cole on Severino's anatomy of *sepia*, or cuttlefish: "His cerebrum may have been a part of the whole of the viscero-pedal system, the lungs are the posterior salivary glands, the first stomach is probably a part of the liver, the ink-sac is confused with the rectum, the second stomach and appendage are the stomach and caecum, the cornua uteri are the ctenidia [part of the respiratory system], the testes (previously regarded as the kidneys) are the branchial hearts, the gall-bladder is the vas deferens and the liver is the testis."[5] Such are the perils of comparative anatomy.

The seventeenth century witnessed fresh reflections and concerns about the demarcation between humans and animals, a key problem because of religious and medical reasons: René Descartes, for example, located the site of the soul in the pineal gland. His claim led anatomists like Thomas Willis and Nicolaus Steno to search for a similar structure in other animals and eventually to question Descartes's views: the pineal gland can be found in other animals, such as fish, which seem devoid of higher functions, and its connections to the rest of the body is similar in different animals and does not justify any special role Descartes attributed to it. The Dutch anatomist Anton Nuck even wrote an obituary to the pineal gland as the site of the soul—echoing Thomas Bartholin's obituary to the liver, in the aftermath of the discovery of the thoracic duct that bypassed it and seemed to deprive it of its hæmatopoietic or blood-making role. Similar concerns involved the organs of speech and the structure of the brain as a whole; speech, of course, was another demarcation point between humans and animals, according to Descartes— though admittedly more because of the way it is used than for the mere ability to articulate sounds, something that parrots can do too. Around 1700 in London Edward Tyson dissected a recently imported "orangutan" in order to locate fundamental differences with our brain: these investigations point to renewed attention to the anatomical basis for our special place in creation.[6]

---

[5] Cole, *Comparative Anatomy*, 141.

[6] Nicolaus Steno, *Lecture on the Anatomy of the Brain*. Introduction by Gustav Scherz (Copenhagen, 1965). Domenico Bertoloni Meli, *Mechanism, Experiment, Disease* (Bal-

An area that became especially significant with the new emphasis on the microstructure of organs of the seventeenth century was the so-called "microscope of nature." Anatomists of the Schaffhausen school, such as Johann Conrad Peyer and Johann Conrad Brunner, referred to the variability in the size of organs and body parts across species as a microscope provided by nature, as if nature had provided the investigator with a microscope by moving from species to species. This strategy did not necessarily involve larger animals; paradoxically, the useful animals could be quite small, what mattered was that the relevant organs would make a given feature more visible. Peyer identified some structures in the intestine and studied them in chickens, where they were especially large, "as if magnified by a microscope." Malpighi's quotations in my introduction above about nature's constant way of operating, method, and necessity are related to such concerns: he argued that since nature's way of operating was uniform, it was legitimate to move from species to species searching for the simplest and most accessible example to unlock her secrets. His belief in this method was so strong that he devoted himself to the study of plants in the hope that their simpler structure may help unlock secrets pertaining to animals; his largest work is *Anatome plantarum* (London, 1675–1679), but already in his first publication, *Epistolae de pulmonibus* of 1661, Malpighi adopted an explanation of their purpose proposed by Borelli and based on the analogy with grafting. As Luigi Belloni has pointed out, the *Epistolae* are a classic example of the "microscope of nature" with regard to the anastomoses of arteries and veins: studying the lungs of frogs and turtles enabled him to close the circle of Harvey's circulation by claiming that blood always flows inside vessels. Such anastomoses are harder to see in higher animals, where the capillary structure is much finer; however, Malpighi argued that it was sufficient for nature to arrange for blood to flow inside vessels and to join their extremities in a net even once to make it probable that the same would happen in other cases too, such as the bladder of frogs; Malpighi would have needed examples from higher animals, where the capillary network was too fine for his microscopes, but lacking that, he had recourse to an analogy from the living world, specifically plants, namely

---

timore, 2011), 79, 166. Richard Serjeantson, "The Passions and Animal Language, 1540-1700," *Journal of the History of Ideas*, 62 (2001), 425-44.

the network of the vessels on leaves. Malpighi was not the first to have recourse to such techniques: Claudius Auberius (died 1658) had dissected the testicle of a wild boar in the mating season in order to see a larger version of structures which are also present in the human testicle, and Massa in the previous century had already relied on a bull in the mating season for similar purposes. Similar techniques are routinely used in recent biological investigations, but Massa and Auberius had relied both on a different species and on a particular time of the year in order to magnify the object of study.[7]

At the same time, in his investigations Malpighi encountered striking and totally unpredictable features. Insects play an especially instructive role in this regard, revealing surprises at every turn: their mode of reproduction, for example, was unclear, and many at the time still believed in spontaneous generation on the assumption that their internal structure would be very simple. In his study of insects and especially the silkworm, Malpighi found female and male genitalia, an elaborate apparatus for producing eggs, and even attempted artificial insemination by coating the eggs with sperm; his work established striking parallels between insects and other animals in an area like generation that was previously thought to involve profound differences. In addition, Malpighi proved that insects breathe and identified in the silkworm nine apertures on each side connected by vessels running inside the body of the insect; his findings highlighted striking similarities in the operations of very different animals and at the same time pointed to startling differences going in the opposite direction, one challenging uniformity: insects lacked lungs, for example, and while investigating their circulatory system, Malpighi identified a long tube with a series of enlargements, which he considered as little hearts. Further, he discovered the periodic reversal in the direction of the heartbeat at different stages of development of the silkworm, from the tail toward the head, then the other way around. These were surprising and unpredictable features; clearly Malpighi's belief in

---

[7] Bertoloni Meli, *Mechanism*, 156. Marcello Malpighi, *Opere Scelte*, edited by Luigi Belloni (Turin, 1967), 24-25; *Opera omnia*, 2 vols., (London, 1686), 2: 143. Niccolò Massa, *Liber introductorius anatomiae*, in Levi Robert Lind, *Pre-Vesalian Anatomy* (Philadelphia, 1975), 199b. Marco Piccolino, "Il nervo, l'alcol e la miccia. Le lunghe strade dell'elettrofisiologia del Novecento," in Marco Piccolino, ed. *Neuroscienze controverse. Da Aristotele alla moderna scienza del linguaggio* (Turin, 2008), 208-48, at 243.

the uniformity of nature could not be applied blindly but had to be carefully monitored at each step to avoid pitfalls.[8]

We can gain a more precise sense of Malpighi's views and worries from his contrast with the Jesuit naturalist Filippo Buonanni over the generation of snails. The initial dispute touched on the topic of spontaneous generation, which was defended by Buonanni, but then it moved to methodological issues: Buonanni defended a radical empiricist position and questioned the method of induction, arguing that not all stars are fixed, since planets move, and not all birds fly, as the ostrich never leaves the ground. Malpighi expressed his dislike for Buonanni's views—and later versions of them—which in his opinion corrupted the true method of philosophizing, making everything uncertain and at the same time every bizarre thing plausible. Indeed, Buonanni had challenged a key tenet of Malpighi's philosophy: the uniformity of nature underpinned many of Malpighi's investigations across different species. To be sure, Malpighi accepted surprising results, but only when they were supported by strong empirical data; generally he would stick to the uniformity of nature unless he was compelled by overwhelming evidence. Others too raised questions about nature's uniformity: up to what extent could one draw conclusions about the human liver from the liver of a snail, or a lizard, or a cricket, or a silkworm, argued Fredrik Ruysch in challenging Malpighi? Thus variability or differences among species offered opportunities through the microscope of nature, but also posed a threat to hasty generalizations.[9]

The situation for believers in the uniformity of nature became especially problematic in the decades around 1700 with regard to the problem of generation. By and large, by the 1660s spontaneous generation had been pushed to the edge of mainstream views by Francesco Redi's sophisticated control experiments on putrefaction. While plants were understood to reproduce from seed, the role of sexual reproduction in the vegetable world was at best unclear and arguably terms like "female" and

---

[8] Malpighi, *De bombyce*, in *Opera*, 2: 1-44. Cole, *Comparative Anatomy*, 183-97, at 196.

[9] Michela Fazzari, "Redi, Buonanni, e la controversia sulla generazione spontanea: una rilettura," in Walter Bernardi and Luigi Guerrini, eds., *Francesco Redi. Un protagonista della scienza moderna* (Florence, 1999), 97-127. Herman Boerhaave and Frederik Ruysch, *Opusculum anatomicum de fabrica glandularum in corpore humano, continens binas episotlas* (Leiden, 1722), 30-31, 68-69. Bertoloni Meli, *Mechanism*, 255-56, 303-5.

"male" for fertile and infertile flowers were used metaphorically. Animal reproduction, however, was understood in terms of fertilization of a female organism by a male one; fertilization could be internal, as in copulation in humans and other higher animals, or external, as in most cases of fish in water.[10]

Within a few decades matters changed dramatically, especially when Dutch anatomist Jan Swammerdam found snails to be hermaphrodites, thus challenging traditional anthropomorphic views about sexual reproduction: whereas up to that point hermaphrodites were considered to be extremely rare occurrences or even monsters, now hermaphroditism was shown to be the normal form of reproduction for an entire species. Swammerdam also challenged anthropomorphic views about the ruler of the beehive, when he discovered that the alleged "king" had eggs and was therefore a "queen," thus shaking widely held assumptions about social order.[11]

At the end of the seventeenth century, the Tübingen botanist and physician Rudolph Jakob Camerarius found on the basis of a refined series of experiments involving the removal of flower parts—which he significantly if colorfully referred to as "castration" for the removal of male parts—and the isolation of female from male flowers, that plants, much like snails, were mostly hermaphrodites, since in most instances the same flower contained male and female parts; matters were slightly more complicated, however, since in some cases like corn there were separate male and female flowers on the same plant, as the plant was monoecious. In others, like spinach or palms, female and male flowers grew on different plants, as they were dioecious. And in a few, like horsetail, the female flowers surprisingly seemed to be missing altogether. In *De sexu plantarum epistola* (1694) Camerarius drew explicitly on the analogy with snails, citing all the authors who had examined their reproduction, beginning with Swammerdam, in arguing that hermaphrodites were not monsters but normal occurrences in some species. Moreover, he drew a further analogy with fish, to argue that in the same way as "external insemination" occurs in water, or at least water does not prevent fertilization, something similar could occur in air too with pollen. The problem

---

[10] Bertoloni Meli, *Mechanism*, 181-84.
[11] *Ibid.*, 195, 267-69.

of horsetails and the identification of the differences between pollen and spores were left unsolved by Camerarius.[12]

In 1744 the Swiss naturalist Abraham Trembley found that fresh water polyps, once cut in half, grew their missing half back, creating havoc in the learned world and especially among supporters of a mechanistic standpoint, since machines don't behave that way. Finally, another Swiss naturalist, Charles Bonnet, found in the 1740s in a series of careful observations that aphids reproduced through parthenogenesis, namely through asexual reproduction without fertilization by a male, dealing a further blow to anthropomorphic views of sexual reproduction. It was in the aftermath to these findings and to the new sensitivity they engendered around mid-century that the French anatomist Pierre Tarin, author of many articles for the *Encyclopédie*, came to question whether anastomoses between arteries and veins could be found also in humans and higher animals, since they had been seen by Antoni van Leeuwenhoek only—he claimed—in fish and frogs, which are cold-blooded animals whose heart has only one ventricle. Later in the century Lazzaro Spallanzani detected anastomoses in chick embryos; a detailed account of the changing fortunes of anastomoses from Malpighi to Spallanzani, as opposed to the sketch offered here, would be a desideratum.[13]

The case of generation highlights at the same time the diversity of nature but also the emergence of striking and totally unpredicted similarities providing novel opportunities for investigation: in the dissolution of the notion of uniformity in nature, new patterns and analogies emerged in wildly different domains. While clearly hasty generalizations from one species to another on matters of generation proved problematic, pondered generalizations opened new horizons of research and conceptualization: it was the explicit recognition that hermaphroditism was a common occurrence in some species such as snails that led Cam-

---

[12] Rudolph Jakob Camerarius, *De sexu plantarum epistola* (Tübingen, 1694). German translation by Martin Möbius, *Ueber das Geschlecht der Pflanzen* (Leipzig, 1899). Bertoloni Meli, *Mechanism*, 267-69.

[13] Thomas L. Hankins, *Science and the Enlightenment* (Cambridge, 1985), 131-33. Marc J. Ratcliff, *The Quest for the Invisible. Microscopy in the Enlightenment* (Farnham, 2009), ch. 5. Pierre Tarin, "Anastomose," in Denis Diderot and Jean le Rond d'Alembert, eds. *Encyclopédie*, vol. I (Paris, 1751), 407b-408°. Lazzaro Spallanzani, *Edizione nazionale delle opere* (Modena, 1984–), part IV, 2: 35-44, 327-35.

erarius to the realization that most plants are hermaphrodites too; similarly, it was the explicit recognition that external fertilization occurs in
fish through water that enabled him to argue for external fertilization in
plants through air. Camerarius emerges as a key figure from our perspective, though he was not unique in this regard: it was thanks to a comparative study with oviparous animals that in 1667 Steno, while dissecting
a female shark, identified the so-called "female testicles" in viviparous
animals as ovaries and called the corresponding ducts "oviducts." The
striking novelty of his finding can be appreciated by bearing in mind that
as late as 1651 William Harvey had deemed the "female testicles" as useless for reproduction.[14]

2. Diversity within a Species

Differences did not just affect generalization across species but also
across individuals within the same species. Several historians, most recently Nancy Siraisi, have addressed the issue in Vesalius, for example, at
the time when the small number of bodies an anatomist could dissect in
his career could lead to dangerous generalizations. Even among Vesalius's
earlier contemporaries, Berengario pointed to the amazing variability of
women's uterus in size, texture, and form, while Massa pointed out that
the length of the human intestine could vary considerably from case to
case, or that nature sometimes doubles the temporal muscles "as a freak."
Vesalius's Paris teacher Jacobus Sylvius discussed a new type of diversity
among humans, one associated with the decline of the human race from
antiquity to his own days: he introduced this notion of decay in order to
save some differences that had been detected between Galen's views and
recent anatomical findings. Changing perceptions of the variability
among humans involving different races, differences in social status and
wealth to do with sensibility of the nervous system or of other anatomical parts, or even the possible distinctive features of the criminal as opposed to the sane body constitute a huge area of research that cannot be
addressed in a short paper, though they provide the opportunity for a few
observations. The surgeon and anatomist Realdo Colombo, for example,

---

[14] Matthew Cobb, *Generation. The Seventeenth-Century Scientists Who Unraveled the
Secrets of Sex, Life, and Growth* (New York, 2006), ch. 4.

argued in 1559 that several thieves he had dissected at Padua, Pisa, and Rome lacked a muscle in the hand, thus establishing an intriguing correlation between anatomy and moral character.[15]

As Anita Guerrini has recently argued, the issue of the individual nature of specific specimens was especially prominent in Claude Perrault's *Histoire des animaux*, a project on a number of exotic animals relying on the menagerie of the Sun King in seventeenth-century Paris: Perrault refused to generalize and to go beyond the specific individuals in front of him. Although Perrault's concerns about generalization and the individuation of characteristics of a species may well have been broader, they seem especially appropriate and wise in view of the fact that he was often dealing with virtually unique specimens of a lion, a chameleon, or a beaver, for example: we face here a situation similar to that faced by early anatomists who had so few human bodies at their disposal that any peculiarity they encountered may have generated problems.[16]

Curiously, in the seventeenth century Willis still accepted the existence of the *rete mirabile* in humans, but only in those "of a slender wit" or "destitute of all force and ardor of the mind." We see here a case of variability both across different species and within the same species, with some humans resembling some animal species, in that slender witted humans can be seen to exhibit anatomical features of some animals, at least in some respects.[17] Sexual differences too may follow under this category, depending on whether women were seen as the other half of the human species, on an equal standing as men, or, following Aristotle, as imperfect men, due to their alleged lack of heat or other imperfections. Tom Laqueuer has argued that at some point during the long eighteenth century views shifted from a hierarchical structure with men at the top

---

[15] William L. Strauss, Jr. and Owsei Temkin, "Vesalius and the Problem of Variability," *Bulletin of the History of Medicine*, 14 (1943), 609-33. Nancy Siraisi, "Vesalius and Human Diversity in '*De humani corporis fabrica*'," *Journal of the Warburg and Courtauld Institutes*, 57 (1994), 60-88. Realdo Colombo, *De re anatomica* (Venice, 1559), 157. Massa, *Liber introductorius*, in Lind, *Pre-Vesalian Anatomy*, 189b, 190b, 193b, 232b. Park, *Secrets of Women*, 181. French, *Dissection and Vivisection*, 136-37, 204.

[16] Guerrini, "The King's Animals," 391.

[17] Thomas Willis, *De cerebro*, transl. Samuel Pordage, in *Of the Anatomy of the Brain and the Description and Use of the Nerves*, in *The Remaining Works of Dr. Thomas Willis* (London, 1681), 85-86.

and women just below, to one in which men and women appear as the equivalent male and female versions of humans. Laqueur's account, however, would benefit from a more careful chronological outline and from taking into account parallel developments about animal and plant generation.[18]

Of course, the fundamental differences between males and females involved the process and organs of generation, whose understanding underwent drastic changes in the seventeenth century: the human uterus seemingly stopped behaving in such erratic ways as the ancients had believed, migrating inside the female body. Other matters about sexual differences were reframed according to the new chemical and mechanical understanding of the body that became predominant in the seventeenth century: the purpose of menstruation in women, for example, was to discard excessively acid and salty particles in blood. In this regard female and male bodies worked differently in health and in disease: a defect of menstruation, for example, led to those acid and salty particles to infect blood and to diseases in the organs of the entire body. Thus female and male pathologies differed beyond specific differences related to the genital parts and child bearing, since an affection in the lungs or brain of a woman could ultimately originate from a defect in menstruation. As Gianna Pomata has reminded us, however, loss of blood in men was at times described in terms similar to those employed for menstruation, thus potentially blurring what may have seemed an obvious distinction.[19]

The sixteenth and seventeenth centuries saw the publication of several *centuriae* of remarkable and unusual cases, whether healthy or diseased; many pertained to teratology. Within the prevailing mechanistic

---

[18] Thomas Laqueur, *Making Sex: Body and Gender from the Greeks to Freud* (Cambridge, MA, 1990).

[19] A critical exam of Plato's views on the wondering womb is in Mark J. Adair, "Plato's View on the 'Wandering Uterus'," *The Classical Journal*, 91 (1996), 153-63. Shirley Roe, *Matter, Life, and Generation: Eighteenth-Century Embryology and the Haller-Wolff Debate* (Cambridge, 1981). For matters pertaining to generation I refer to Karin J. Ekholm, *Generation and its Problems: Harvey, Highmore, and Their Contemporaries* (Ph.D. thesis, Indiana University, Bloomington, 2011). See also Gianna Pomata, "Menstruating Men: Similarity and Difference of the Sexes in Early Modern Medicine," in *Generation and Degeneration: Tropes of Reproduction in Literature and History from Antiquity through Early Modern Europe*, ed. Valeria Finucci and Kevin Brownlee (Durham, NC, 2001), 109-52.

framework of the time, monsters proved especially helpful and revealing: whereas in the Renaissance they were often taken as portentous signs to be deciphered at times in religious, political, or medical contexts, announcing reforms, upheavals, and epidemics, in the seventeenth century they were seen as the products of the same laws applying to normal cases; in fact, precisely because the laws at play were the same but the outcome could be dramatically different, they were seen as potentially revealing of the inner workings of nature. Malpighi made such claims explicit when he stated: "Monsters and other mistakes dissipate our ignorance more easily and reliably than the remarkable and polished machines of Nature." While working in unusual ways, nature was more likely to reveal her secrets.[20]

Thus, much as in the case of the diversity among species, also individual variability and even monsters posed a challenge to generalizations while at the same time presenting an opportunity for further reflections and investigations: an unusual case may lead to error in hasty generalizations, but may also help unlock the secrets of nature.

3. Diversity within an Organism

But there is a further level of diversity that we must consider, one that is quite complex and problematic in its own right. The same body can differ significantly depending on age, season of the year, time of the month, and even geographical location, for example. Such variations posed problems not only in moving from one individual to another but also for the very same individual, in that the anatomical features observed in certain circumstances may not be found in others. This issue was well known since antiquity, and renaissance anatomists were well aware of it when they sought to dissect a middle-aged (usually male) body at public functions. Cartilages, bones, and muscles could vary considerably depending on age, and the same body could differ also depending on whether it is in a hot and dry or cold and wet climate, such as in winter or summer, or on the phase of the reproductive cycle, menstrual cycle for women or broadly corresponding stages for non-human animals: we encounter

---

[20] Domenico Bertoloni Meli, "Blood, Monsters, and Necessity in Malpighi's *De polypo cordis*," *Medical History*, 45 (2001), 511-22, at 518.

here another instance of variability related to sexual differences, after different modes of reproduction and differences between male and female bodies. Nor are female animals the only examples of variability in relation to a sexual cycle: we have seen above that both Massa and Auberius dissected the testicles of a bull and a wild boar, respectively, during the mating season, in order to uncover their structure at a time when all the parts were especially enlarged and distended. Lastly, certain body parts could differ depending on when the animals had eaten, as the Pavia anatomist Gasparo Aselli realized when he searched for the milky vein—or the vessels carrying digested food away from the intestine—in a dog and found none: only in a dog that had been fed a few hours before were such ephemeral vessels visible. Although Aselli was able in this way to provide a detailed analysis of the milky veins, the technique he employed was not new: Galen had already used it long before.[21]

Individual variability had therapeutic implications as well in that remedies appropriate for a given age, sex, temperament, season, and geographical location, could be inadequate in different circumstances. Standard medical consultations on patients, for example, start by specifying precisely these features: the remedies for an old or young man or woman would differ, and the cure for a recurrent disease of the same individual would not remain unchanged as that individual aged. Would the cures appropriate for a European in Europe be the same for the same individual in Africa or America? We witness here the problematic connection between anatomy and medical practice discussed in the opening of this essay.

Since my work concerns plants as well, it is worth remembering that seasonal and climatic changes in the vegetable world can of course be huge. The botanist Giovanni Battista Trionfetti, prefect of the Botanic Gardens at La Sapienza University in Rome, and a friend of Buonanni's, argued in the 1670s that moving a plant from the wild to a protected environment and vice versa, or changing its living conditions, may not only change the plant's size but also induce metamorphosis, which he claimed he had observed in wheat changing into darnel. We find here that changes of an individual specimen made it cross species, if one believes Trionfetti.[22]

---

[21] Gasparo Aselli, *De lactibus* (Milan, 1627), 20. Galen, *On the Natural Faculties*, III, 4.
[22] Betoloni Meli, *Mechanism*, 256-59.

There is yet another aspect associated with generalizing knowledge in the context of a single organism. We have seen that the same organ in animals of different species may differ in size and enable investigation in the most favorable case, so that knowledge could be transferred to other cases. Something similar happened in generalizing results from one organ or body part to other organs or body parts within the same organism: differences in size provided the opportunity to unlock nature's secrets. Once again, Massa is quite useful in this regard, when he states that optic nerves seem to be perforated in large animals, "which reason also persuades us to believe is the case in all other nerves so that their power may be carried down through them." We find here the same form of double generalization both across species and across the very same organism, moving from the optic nerve to other nerves. Massa was by no means the only one to draw such generalizations. Malpighi, for example, could observe the anastomoses between arteries and veins only in the lungs of certain animals, such as frogs and turtles: he then generalized this result not only to the lungs of other animals but also to other organs and body parts of the same animal as well, where the fine capillary network was not visible with the instruments at his disposal. Thus the view that blood always flows inside vessels was based on a rather thin body of evidence, as Pierre Tarin was to point out quite acutely in 1751. Also in the case of the micro-structures or glomerules—the sites of the separation of urine—Malpighi found in the kidneys, for example, he relied on generalization and analogy when he identified the glomerules as glandular. Glands, however, have an afferent artery, an efferent vein, and also a nervous termination, which he could not detect in the glomerules; thus he inferred by analogy with other glands in the body that the glomerules too have a nervous termination. We witness here a puzzling inference from the general structure of a body part (glands) to the specific structure of that part in an organ (the glomerules in the kidneys).[23]

Thus variability and changes within the same organism too raised both epistemological and practical problems: in the cases of Massa and Malpighi the very same technique gave contrasting results. Within the time covered by my work, nerves were shown not to be perforated after

---

[23] Malpighi, *Opera omnia*, 2: 141-43, 92, 173. Massa, *Liber introductorius*, in Lind, *Prevesalian Anatomy*, 240b.

all and the existence of anastomoses between arteries and veins was questioned.

Conclusion

Starting from the beginning of the sixteenth century, we detect a growing awareness of diversity and variability in nature at many levels, among species, within a species, and even within a single organism. The empirical realization that nature is so variable and complex posed problems about which anatomists showed considerable epistemological and methodological sophistication already from the 1520s, witness Berengario's emphasis on differences and variability at all levels, both among species with regard to the *rete mirabile* and among organisms with regard to the size of the uterus, for example; Massa's frequent discussions of techniques and variability, with regard to differences in length of the human intestine, for example, and the appearance of freak muscles; Vesalius's boastful emphasis on human as opposed to animal dissection and his challenge to Galen; Colombo's peculiar claim about the lack of a muscle in the hand of thieves; and Fabricius's broad focus on *anatomia comparata*.

Diversity and variability were exploited by anatomists who moved across species and organisms in order to find the most effective and suitable specimen to unlock nature's secrets: the expression "microscope of nature" captures the efforts by a number of scholars such as Auberius, Peyer, and Malpighi in studying wild boar's testicles, chickens' intestines, frogs' and turtles' lungs. Over a century earlier, however, Massa had already exploited the size of testicles in different species and within the same organism in normal circumstances and at mating time, for example, and the size and structure of optic nerves, which enabled him to generalize to other nerves. The notion of the uniformity of nature provided a crucial philosophical underpinning to those investigations.

With the problem of reproduction the notion of the uniformity of nature met a set of seemingly insurmountable challenges: it just seemed impossible to harness the strikingly different behavior of snails, bees, corn, spinach, palms, fish, horsetail, fresh water polyps, and aphids. It was in the aftermath of startling findings on generation that Pierre Tarin questioned the general occurrence of anastomoses between arteries and veins.

Yet within these empirical observations on a bewildering range of organisms there wasn't just growing chaos: Steno's findings about structural parallels between oviparous and viviparous animals led him to identify the so-called "female testicles" as ovaries and name the Fallopian tubes "oviducts," while Malpighi identified genitalia and eggs in insects. Further, while what we have called the anthropomorphic mode of reproduction collapsed, new, entirely unpredictable patterns emerged: Camerarius stands out as a key figure in my story, in that he was able to identify those new patterns from a composite set of data, from Swammerdam's findings about the hermaphroditism of snails to the reproduction of plants, and from the fertilization of fish eggs in water to plant fertilization through the atmosphere. Snails and fishes became the unlikely exemplars underpinning his claims about sexual reproduction in plants and marking the emergence of a new pluralistic order in our understanding of nature and especially of reproduction, one that was by no means settled in a definitive way, witness his bewilderment at the lack of female horsetail.

III. RELEVANCE OF CASE STUDIES

Experiment, Observation, Self-observation. Empiricism and the 'Reasonable Physicians' of the Early Enlightenment

Carsten Zelle
*Ruhr-Universität Bochum**

Abstract

This article aims to analyze the mechanisms of empirical data collection in medicine and psychology in the early Enlightenment by means of experiment, observation and self-observation, while associating them with their discursive forms of representation; namely, the case narrative. The combination of empirical and discursive anthropo-techniques leads to explanations on the anthro*poietics* of the Enlightenment; i.e., the question of how the habitus of man was shaped around 1750. Texts of four German 'reasonable physicians' will be considered: Friedrich Hoffmann (1660–1742), Johann Gottlieb Krüger (1715–1759), Andreas Elias Büchner (1701–1769) and Johann August Unzer (1727–1799).

Keywords

Andreas Elias Büchner, Christian Wolff, Friedrich Hoffmann, Johann Gottlieb Krüger, Johann August Unzer, anthropology, casus, empirical psychology, empirico-rationalism, *experientia*, experiment, *historia morbi*, observation, poetics of knowledge, ratio, self-observation

Introduction

The theme of this article arose in the context of research into literary anthropology in the eighteenth century, which initially focused on a group of 'reasonable physicians' at the Prussian reform university of Halle/Saale. Having overcome Cartesian dualism of substance, philo-

* Ruhr-Universität Bochum, Germanistisches Institut, Universitätsstraße 150, 44780 Bochum, Germany (carsten.zelle@rub.de). This article has been translated from the German by Julia Lippmann (Bochum).

sophically educated medical scientists such as Johann Gottlob Krüger (1715–1759) or Johann August Unzer (1727–1799) expanded their perspective to focus on the 'whole man'. They were hence the forerunners of a new medico-philosophical approach, which formed the basis of the Commercium-Anthropology of the 'philosophical physicians' of the late Enlightenment (e.g., Ernst Platner and Friedrich Schiller, to name just two).[1] Such aspects of an anthropology or empirical psychology, which is centered around the 'whole man' have since that time been replaced by literary-scientific or 'poetological' questions of the discursive representation of anthropological or rather psychological knowledge, especially in the prose genre of the case narrative (e.g., the medical history or *historia morbi*).[2] Departing from the terminology that is commonly used in the relevant specialist literature, I shall here not refer to 'case reports', 'case stories', 'case descriptions' or 'case studies' but rather to case *narratives*.[3] The terminological choice helps to indicate the historiographical difference between event and story and to take into account the narratological distinction between *histoire* and *récit*.

In this context, 'poetics of knowledge' characterizes an approach that takes into account the discursive representation of knowledge or science, respectively. That means that it analyzes the types of texts in which knowledge is represented and the kinds of ways in which scientific texts are referred to, which metaphors are being used and which rhetorical strategies are employed to create evidence and effects of truth. Thus, questions of the intrinsic laws of expository texts, of narratology, metaphorology and rhetoric shall play a significant role. The question of how knowledge, and also 'scientific knowledge', is represented, the 'poetics of knowledge' confronts one with the observation that a so-called *factum* is not simply 'given', but rather—in compliance with Latin etymology— is something that is 'created'. According to Greek etymology, the 'poetics

---

[1] Carsten Zelle, "Zur Idee des 'ganzen Menschen' im 18. Jahrhundert," in Udo Sträter, ed., *Die „Neue Kreatur"—Pietismus und Anthropologie. Beiträge zum II. Internationaler Kongress für Pietismusforschung 2005*, vol. I (Halle and Tübingen, 2008), 45-61.

[2] Carsten Zelle, "'Die Geschichte bestehet in einer Erzählung'. Poetik der medizinischen Fallerzählung bei Andreas Elias Büchner (1701–1769)," *Zeitschrift für Germanistik*, 19/2 (2009), 301-16.

[3] Cf. Stefan Willer, "Fallgeschichte," in Bettina Jagow and Florian Steger, eds., *Literatur und Medizin. Ein Lexikon* (Göttingen, 2005), 231-35.

of knowledge' in its strong form is hence *'poietics* of knowledge'; i.e., an approach that focuses on the question of how scientific facts are generated.[4]

This article aims to analyze the mechanisms of empirical data collection in medicine and psychology in the early Enlightenment by means of experiment, observation and self-observation, while associating it with its discursive forms of representation; namely, the *casus*, the expository text form of the case narrative. The combination of empirical and discursive anthropo-techniques—i.e., techniques that pertain to man and the knowledge of man—leads to some explanations of the anthro*poietics* of the Enlightenment. In fact, I shall be interested in the question of how the habitus of man was shaped around 1750.[5]

These investigations are divided into three sections:

1) Friedrich Hoffmann's medical empirico-rationalism: *experientia* and *ratio*. In this context, we will study the preambles to the twelve volumes of *Medicina Consultatoria* by Halle medical scientist Friedrich Hoffmann (1660–1742). The collection comprises 610 *casus*, case reports, which were published between 1721 and 1739. Each volume, except for the last, one includes a preamble. The 11 preambles provide a comprehensive overview of Hoffmann's medical approach and its foundations.

2) Experiment, observation, self-observation: in this section, I will focus on the methods of empirical data collection on the basis of observations and experiments—an approach that was showcased by 'reasonable physician' Johann Gottlieb Krüger in the introduction to his *Attempt at an Experimental Psychology* (1765). It was further illustrated by Andreas Elias Büchner (1701–1769) in his work *The Reasonably Guessing and Successfully Curing Medicus* (1762/65), in a chapter specifically dedicated to the rules "one should observe when conducting medical experiments."

3) 'Reforging' man—the anthro*poietics* of the 'reasonable physicians': In the third and last section of this article we will turn to a brief instruction by Johann August Unzer that was published in his educational

---

[4] Cf. Joseph Vogl, "Für eine Poetologie des Wissens," in Karl Richter, Jörg Schönert and Michael Titzmann, eds., *Die Literatur und die Wissenschaften 1770–1930* (Stuttgart 1997), 107-27.

[5] Carsten Zelle, "Klopstocks Reitkur—Zur Konkurrenz christlicher Lebensordnung und weltlicher Diät um 1750," in Michael Hofmann and Carsten Zelle, eds., *Aufklärung und Religion—Neue Perspektiven* (Hannover 2010), 65-84.

journal *The Physician* (1759–1764). In the 9th and 160th pieces the Altona medical scientist repeatedly tried to convey to his patient the method of self-observation and its documentation in written form.

1.　Friedrich Hoffmann's Medical Empirico-rationalism: *experientia* and *ratio*

In the preamble to the first volume of his *Natural Sciences* (1740), Johann Gottlob Krüger uses a special rhetorical strategy to justify his enterprise given that from Aristotle's times to the present, many similar papers had been published. Krüger, professor of philosophy and medicine, emphasizes the innovative quality that distinguishes his *Natural Sciences* from older works, which over time had become obsolete. As Krüger claims, "for about 50 years the natural sciences have been gaining a different shape." Dramatically, he refers to a break in the history of science: an 'empirico-rationalist turn'. Hence the numerous old books that "merely consisted of empty words and sweet dreams" did not deserve "to be called observations of nature." As opposed to the old knowledge, which is reduced to mere speculation, Krüger utilizes the persuasive means of a new era: reason and experience. Krüger explains the methodical concepts, which have been giving natural science its new shape since the turn of the eighteenth century as follows:

> One does not acknowledge any physical approach anymore that is not built on reason and experience as the most solid columns of all human knowledge. Thus one dares not claim anything that cannot be proven on the basis of correct reasonable conclusions or accurately conducted experiments and observations.

In short, as Krüger sums up, "one seeks to maintain reason and experience in a constant agreement."[6] Somewhat later, Krüger associates the continuous agreement between empiricism and *ratio* with the 'mathe-

---

6) Johann Gottlob Krüger, *Naturlehre*, part I: *Physik* [1. ed. 1740]. 5. ed. (Halle 1771), b^r f. („Nur seit etwa 50. Jahren hat die Naturlehre eine andere Gestalt bekommen. Man will keinen physicalischen Lehrbegriff mehr gelten lassen, der nicht auf Vernunft und Erfahrung, als die festesten Grundsäulen aller menschlichen Erkenntniß, gebauet ist. Man getrauet sich daher nichts zu behaupten, was man nicht durch richtige Vernunftschlüsse, oder sorgfältig angestellte Experimente und Observationen beweisen kan.

matical approach', comparing the philosophers who follow it to elephants "that never move their second foot forward before the first one stands rather firmly."[7]

The empirico-rationalist epistemology that Krüger refers to here follows the principles laid down by Christian Wolff (1679–1754), which have been championed in medicine, first and foremost, by Friedrich Hoffmann (1660–1742), a teacher of Krüger's. Krüger ascribes to Wolff's mathematical method the fact that, instead of "obscure concepts and unfounded opinions, distinctness and thoroughness" were prevailing.[8] Furthermore, he justifies the application of empirical approaches in psychology, citing Wolff's statement, "that it would be far easier to explore the soul if one could discover the true texture of the human brain through appropriate magnifying glasses."[9] The empirico-rationalist scientific approach is equally pursued by the 'reasonable physicians' and Christian Wolff, who founded his natural-scientific research on observations and experiments. In addition, he tried to merge accurate reason and thorough experience in his epistemology and emphasized how important it was not to assume anything "which cannot be proven by infallible experiences."[10]

Hoffmann too builds his medical epistemology on reason and experience, records his *observationes* in the form of a *historia morbi* and outlines the principles of his nosology and the fundamentals of therapy. In

---

Kurtz, man sucht Vernunft und Erfahrung in einer beständigen Uebereinstimmung zu erhalten.")

[7] Krüger, *Naturlehre*, part II: *Physiologie* [1. ed. 1743]. 2. ed. (Halle 1748), "Vorrede," b6ᵛ f. („Denn ich habe mir sagen lassen, die wahren Philosophen müßten wie die Elephanten seyn, welche niemals den andern Fuß fortsetzen, ehe der erstere recht feste stehet.")

[8] Krüger, *Physiologie*, 188 („Wie sehr muß man also nicht dem Herrn Cantzler von Wolffen verbunden seyn, der die mathematische Methode mit so gutem Fortgange in die Weltweisheit eingeführet hat, daß nunmehr Deutlichkeit und Gründlichkeit, die Wissenschaften mit Erklärungen und Beweisthümern erfüllet, an deren Stelle man bey denen Alten kaum etwas anders als dunckele Begriffe und ungegründete Meinungen antrift.").

[9] Krüger, *Naturlehre*, part III.1: *Pathologie*, part. III.2: *Besondere Pathologie* (Halle 1750), 516.

[10] Christian Wolff, *Allerhand nützliche Versuche, dadurch zu genauer Erkäntniß der Natur und Kunst der Weg gebähnet wird* […]. *Erster Theil* [1. ed. 1721]. 4. ed. (Halle 1745), „Vorrede,")(7ʳ. See Günter Mühlpfordt, "Die organischen Naturwissenschaften in Wolffs empiriorationalistischer Enzyklopädistik," *Il cannocchiale*, 2.3 (1989), 77-106.

view of *"praeservation"*—i.e., *preventative* health care, to which he attaches special importance—he emphasizes the significance of diet and one's lifestyle.[11] According to Hoffmann, the "maintenance" and "restoration of health" is the *"finis* of *medicine."*[12] He repeats this over and over again; e.g., in his preamble to volume I: "On the Excellent Use of *Observationum* and *Consiliorum Medicorum"* Hoffmann insists over and over that the conjunction between *"experientia* and *ratio"* is the foundation of 'reasonable' medicine. To him observation and documentation in a complete *historia morbi* are the ultimate prerequisites of medical progress that had so far been lacking.[13] Practical medicine should rest upon two fundamentals: "Firstly, comprehensively and meticulously described *Casus, Observationes* and *Morborum historiæ*, of which there were unfortunately only a few. The other *fundament* consists of a *solid theory."* The "main *fundament*," however, are "thorough *observations."*[14] Within the empirico-rationalist interplay Hoffmann prioritizes induction insofar as he subordinates the *"veritates intellectuales"* to the *"veritates historicae."* At the same time, he sees the progress of physics "solely achieved on the

---

[11] Friedrich Hoffmann, *Medicina Consultatoria: Worinnen Unterschiedliche über einige schwehre Casus ausgearbeitete Consilia, auch Responsa Facultatis Medicæ enthalten* [...], 12 vols. (Halle 1721–1739), vol. 11, 1738, "Vorrede,")(3ʳ. On the basis of inspection of the Frankfurt copy (University of Frankfurt, Senckenberg Institute for the History and Ethics of Medicine, Ges.med. 89 1721/1, vols. 1–10) and the Düsseldorf copy (Sign. Med. I 487, 12 vols.) of *Medicina Consultatoria*, it would appear that there must exist at least two prints with roughly the same content. The two copies, however, differ in using virgule (Frankfurt copy) resp. comma (Düsseldorf copy) and in respect of the page breaks. This article is based on the Düsseldorf copy which is easily accessible in digital format.

[12] Hoffmann, *Medicina Consultatoria*, 1, 1721, "Vorrede," („Von dem vortrefflichen Nutzen derer *Observationum* und *Consiliorum Medicorum"*),)()(ᵛ. On Hoffmann's empirico-rationalist method, see Jürgen Helm, "Beobachten, Sammeln, Verallgemeinern. Konzepte und Praktiken zur Herstellung medizinischen Wissens," in Rudolf Behrens and Carsten Zelle, eds., *Der ärztliche Fallbericht. Epistemische Grundlagen und textuelle Strukturen dargestellter Beobachtung* (Wiesbaden 2012), 23-36; and Helm "'observatio' und 'experientia'—Fallgeschichten in der Medizin des 18. Jahrhunderts," in Christian Soboth and Udo Sträter, eds., *"Aus Gottes Wort und eigener Erfahrung gezeiget." Erfahrung—Glauben, Erkennen und Handeln im Pietismus. Beiträge zum III. Internationaler Kongress für Pietismusforschung 2009*, vol. I (Halle 2012), 361-75.

[13] Hoffmann, *Medicina Consultatoria*, 1, 1721, "Vorrede,")()(ʳ.

[14] *Ibid.*, 4, 1724, "Vorrede,"):(2ᵛ.

basis of diligent *observationes* and *experimenta*," leaving in no doubt the
fact "that in *Medicine experienz* was superordinate to all *raisonnement*."[15]

In view of recent research into the forms and functions of medical case
reports as one of the epistemic genres of the early modern era, it might
seem at first surprising that Hoffmann keeps on complaining about the
lack of medical *"progressus*."[16] Instead, there were uncertainty, doubt,
discrepant opinions, dissent and controversy among medical scientists.
Hoffmann sees the reason for this in the fact that "neither in recent nor
in older times sufficient importance had been placed on complete *historias morborum* that were hence only very rarely to be found and not easily to be compiled among all *Scribenten*."[17] Elsewhere, he complains that

> Now [due to the lack of complete and explicit *observationes*; C.Z.] it has almost
> come so far that nearly every school principal has his own *Logic*, a *Superintendens*,
> a *Catechismum* and almost every well-known professor is about to conceive and
> write a peculiar theory that would then comprise of so many *principia* and *hypoth-
> eses* that the youth does not know where to turn to.[18]

---

[15] *Ibid.*, 3, 1723, "Vorrede,"):(3ʳ f. („Die Wissenschaft der natürlichen Dinge, die vor
Alters in bloßen Wörtern bestund, ist eintzig und allein durch fleißige *observationes*
und *experimenta* [...] in guten Stand gekommen.") and):(4ᵛ („Denn wer kan wohl in
einigen Zweifel ziehen, daß in der *Medicin* die *experienz* allen *raisonnement* vorgehe?")

[16] See Johanna Geyer-Kordesch, "Medizinische Fallbeschreibungen und ihre Bedeu-
tung in der Wissensreform des 17. und 18. Jahrhunderts," *Medizin, Gesellschaft, Geschichte.
Jahrbuch des Instituts für Geschichte der Medizin der Robert Bosch-Stiftung*, 9 (1990), 7-19.
Michael Stolberg, "Formen und Funktionen medizinischer Fallberichte in der Frühen
Neuzeit (1500–1800)," in Johannes Süßmann, Susanne Schulz, and Gisela Engel, eds.,
Fallstudien. Theorie—Geschichte—Methode (Berlin 2007), 81-95; Gianna Pomata, "Shar-
ing Cases: The *Observationes* in Early Modern Medicine," *Early Science and Medicine*, 15
(2010), 193-236.

[17] Hoffmann, *Medicina Consultatoria*, 1, 1721, "Vorrede,")()()(3ᵛ: "weil man sich weder
zu den alten, noch zu den neuen Zeiten genugsam auf vollständige *historias morborum*
geleget, die gewiß bey allen *Scribenten* sehr spahrsam zu finden und zusammen zu
suchen sind."

[18] *Ibid.*, 3, 1723, "Vorrede,")(4ʳ („Es ist ja leider fast so weit gekommen, daß fast ein
jeglicher Schul=*Rector* seine eigne *Logic*, ein *Superintendens* einen *Catechismum*, also
auch fast ieglicher berühmter *Professor* eine sonderliche *Theorie* formiren und schreiben
will, da denn so vielerley *principia* und *hypotheses* vorkommen, daß die Jugend nicht
weiß, wohin sie sich wenden soll.")

There is hardly a preamble to his collection in which Hoffmann does not blame "the lack of adequate and comprehensive *Observatio*nen" for the unsatisfactory, imperfect state of the "*cognitio medica rationalis.*"[19]

What is the reason for Hoffmann's numerous complaints about the low number of 'accurate' *casus*? Research over the last few years has documented the increase of case story collections since the end of the sixteenth century.[20] Hoffmann could thus have looked back on a comprehensive, well-documented corpus of case reports. It seems that Hoffmann is referring to a special kind of format which concerns both the nature of observation and the manner of its discursive representation.

Medical experience is conceived as an attentive and exhaustive way of observing things and the changes that are related to the human body. "I hence describe the experience in *medicine* as an *attenta & completa observatio* [...]," Hoffmann writes in the preamble that serves as the opening to his collection.[21] An observation is 'attentive' and 'complete' if it follows the norms that Hoffmann defined for their written documentation. The empirical process is classified according to the way it has been documented. Experience and reason, he claims in 1723 in his "Preamble on the Use of Good *Observationum* and the Harm Caused by a Wrong *Theoria in praxi medica*," is hence "the ability to observe and to write."[22] According to Hoffmann, empirical data collection and discursive fixation, observation or experimentation and writing are inseparable and complementary. Hence, the order of things is reversed insofar as the forms and techniques of discursive fixation guide the attention of the empirical scientist. Hoffmann's medical methodology is based on this double imperative demanding "observe, write!" which would characterize the approach of the empirical 'natural scientists' in the later eighteenth century.[23]

---

19) *Ibid.*, 5, 1726, "Vorrede,")(3ᵛ.

20) See, most recently, Gianna Pomata, "Observation Rising: Birth of an Epistemic Genre, ca. 1500–1650," in Lorraine Daston and Elizabeth Lunbeck, eds., *Histories of Scientific Observation* (Chicago, 2011), 45-80.

21) Hoffmann, *Medicina Consultatoria,* 1, 1721, "Vorrede,")()(ᵛ.

22) *Ibid.*, 3, 1723, "Vorrede Von dem Nutzen guter *Observationum* und Schaden der falschen *Theoria in praxi medica*,"):(2ᵛ.

23) Johann Karl Wezel,, "Über die Erziehungsgeschichten," *Pädagogische Unterhand-*

Following Hoffmann's epistemological model, theory and empiricism are correlated to one another. If the theory is lacking experience it is downgraded to mere "speculations,"[24] opening the door for "*Charletaneria medica*."[25] If, on the other hand, observation is lacking theoretical reflection, it becomes mere "unreasonable empiricism and botch."[26] In Hoffmann's opinion, pure, unreflected empiricism has pejorative connotations. According to him, what was important was "not to proceed *empirice*, but *methodice*," since a 'reasonable physician' stood out by his ability to observe and to analyze ("*observiren und meditiren*"). A "*medicus*" thus had the reputation "that he would not cure *empirice* but adhered to the *rationales*," which included a "healthy and active intellect" and the knowledge of the "order of nature."[27]

What distinguished the previous cases that were documented in the early modern period from Hoffmann's *casus* of the early Enlightenment were "accurate and complete *observations*,"[28] which were brought to light in a clear, comprehensible and well-written manner.[29] Furthermore Hoffmann highlights the older practice of inventing *casus* that were documented in the *casualia collegia* to support "construed *hypotheses*," arguing that such a method would be good-for-nothing.[30] Hoffmann compares these books that accumulated "many useless and unfortunately fictitious" observations with other works that included "perfect *observations*" and would hence be worth communicating to "the public."[31]

According to Hoffmann, observation and writing form a recursive system of operations that support and reinforce one another. It is centered around an extensive list of topics that determine the *observatio* (and the semantic field around *casus*) as a concept that comprises of ambiguity, event and narration, all at the same time. The *observatio* or *historia mor-*

---

lungen. Philanthropisches Journal für die Erzieher und das Publicum, 2 (1778/79), 21-43, here 43.

24) Hoffmann, *Medicina Consultatoria*, 3, 1723, "Vorrede,"):(4ᵛ.
25) *Ibid.*, 8, 1731, "Vorrede,")(4ᵛ.
26) *Ibid.*, 4, 1724, "Vorrede,"):(3ʳ.
27) *Ibid.*, 9, 1732, "Vorrede,")(3ʳ f.
28) *Ibid.*, 1, 1721, "Vorrede,")()(2ᵛ.
29) *Ibid.*, 5, 1726, "Vorrede,")(3ʳ.
30) *Ibid.*, 5, 1726, "Vorrede,")()()(2ᵛ.
31) *Ibid.*, 6, 1728, "Vorrede,")(3ᵛ.

bi are comprised of "certain requisitia" that are related to four dimensions: firstly, to the "whole nature" of the patient (*"corporis aegrotanis naturam"*); secondly, to the perfect *historia* (comprising *"morbi originem, causas progressum, symptomata, eventum"*); thirdly, to therapy, the prescribed medication and preventative measures (*"curam, medicamentorum operationem, praeservationem"*); and fourthly—if the illness should ultimately be lethal despite of all medical endeavours—to the autopsy results (*"sectionem defunctorum"*). The overall topic of the "complete and comprehensively described casus" that is developed here was improved by later physicians such as Unzer and Andreas Elias Büchner. It takes up nearly five pages of text.[32]

2. Experiment, Observation, Self-observation

Reading the programmatic preambles to Hoffmann's *Medicina Consultatoria* one learns that in the first half of the eighteenth century, rationalism and empiricism were no competing epistemological models, but, on the contrary, that reason and experience were inseparably linked.[33] The concept was centered around the correlation between an a priori and an a posteriori process of gaining knowledge according to which induction and deduction were inseparable and mutually interdependent. Accordingly, experience had a supportive and regulatory function within the concept formation process while reason served as the key to empirical data collection.[34] Concept formation takes place through ap-

---

[32] *Ibid.,* 1, 1721, "Vorrede,")()(2ᵛ-)()(4ᵛ.

[33] See Wolfgang Röd, *Die Philosophie der Neuzeit*, vol. 2, *Von Newton bis Rousseau* (München, 1984), II, esp. 249 f.; Mühlpfordt, „Die organischen Naturwissenschaften"; Hans Jürgen Engfer, *Empirismus versus Rationalismus. Kritik eines philosophischen Schemas* (Paderborn, 1996), esp. 268-83; Lothar Kreimendahl, "Empiristische Elemente im Denken Christian Wolffs," in Jürgen Stolzenberg and Oliver-Pierre Rudolph, eds., *Christian Wolff und die europäische Aufklärung. Akten des 1. Internationalen Christian Wolff-Kongresses, Halle (Saale), 4.-8. April 2004*, vol. 1: *Plenums- und Abendvorträge* (Hildesheim, Zürich, New York, 2007), 95-112.

[34] See Ernst Cassirer, *Das Erkenntnisproblem in der Philosophie und Wissenschaft der neueren Zeit. Zweiter Band* [1. ed. 1907; 3. ed. 1922], ed. Dagmar Vogel (Hamburg 1999), II, 161, for the foundation of a theory of empirical knowledge in Tschirnhaus's *Medicina mentis* (1687, ²1695), which was to influence Wolff strongly.

prehension; i.e., the entirety of sensual perceptions, conveyed by the external and internal senses. These perceptions were either external things perceived by the five exterior senses (*sensus exteriores: tactus, visus, auditus, olfactus, gustus*) and their technical extensions or internal emotional processes perceived by the *sensus interiores*. This taxonomy of the senses forms the basis to a classification of different *modi* of empirical data collection. In this context, Krüger's work shall serve as the guideline for the analysis of this epistemic concept; namely, his *Versuch einer Experimental=Seelenlehre (Attempt at an Experimental Psychology)*. Published in 1756, this was his last significant work, and it illustrated the underlying empirical methodology in its introduction.[35] Like Hoffmann, Krüger sees empirical knowledge acquisition in the context of of Lutheran pessimism of a postlapsarian anthropology *concerning* knowledge. Hoffmann, for instance, writes about "man who is wretched and thoroughly rotten in soul, body, intellect and mind after the miserable fall of mankind."[36] In short, then, the fall of mankind had shattered man's original epistemic ability. Since then, Krüger argues, the obligation "to learn about the world through experience" has been imposed on man.[37] The "limitations of our intellect" are compensated by "experience, which is actually a realization that one obtained through the senses."[38] The interplay between reason and experience, which were regarded as the "two main columns of human knowledge" by the 'reasonable physicians', is finally decided in favor of empiricism—also from Hoffmann's point of view.[39] Using genealogical metaphors Krüger refers to reason as the

---

[35] See Carsten Zelle, "Experimentalseelenlehre und Erfahrungsseelenkunde. Zur Unterscheidung von Erfahrung, Beobachtung und Experiment bei Johann Gottlob Krüger und Karl Philipp Moritz," in Carsten Zelle, ed., *"Vernünftige Ärzte." Hallesche Psychomediziner und die Anfänge der Anthropologie in der deutschsprachigen Frühaufklärung* (Tübingen, 2001), 173-85.

[36] Hoffmann, *Medicina Consultatoria*, 1, 1721, "Vorrede,")(2ᵛ ("Daß der elende und nach dem kläglichen Sünden=Fall an Seele, Leib, Verstand und Gemüthe gantz verdorbene Mensch [...]").

[37] Johann Gottlob Krüger, *Versuch einer Experimental=Seelenlehre*. [Incl.:] *Anhang verschiedener Wahrnehmungen, welche zur Erläuterung der Seelenlehre dienen*, 2 vols. (Halle and Helmstädt, 1756), § 4, 5.

[38] *Ibid.*, 5 f.

[39] *Ibid.*, § 2, 2. See Andreas Elias Büchner, *Der vernünftig rathende und glücklich curirende Medicus*, 2 vols. (Erfurt, 1762/65); Büchner, *Medicus*, II, 163: "Ein wahrer Arzte muß

"daughter of experience," and to experience as the "mother of reason." At the same time he prioritizes the a posteriori to the a priori method of gaining knowledge, using different literary comparisons to ridicule pure rationalism: "Do not those who are trying merely to follow reason while neglecting all sensual concepts resemble children who are hoping to move just by imitating the carter's speech though sitting in a horseless carriage?" or: "Striving to become a natural scientist without experience means to undertake a journey with blindfolded eyes just to satisfy one's curiosity."[40] Relying on his concept of an empirical psychology—i.e. the endeavour "to explore the soul through experience"—Krüger sees methods ways of data collection, "using the internal and external senses."[41]

While the concept of the 'external senses' is quite obvious, it is difficult to capture what was meant by 'internal sense' in the eighteenth century. In what way one should picture this kind of "epistemic self-reflexion" as a means of empirical data collection it is only mentioned by Krüger in passing, and moreover in a negative context.[42] Although philosophy had, "commendably," only just began along the troublesome path towards the exploration of the psyche through the inner sense, it had "discovered," as Krüger comments ironically, "more than one might be capable of discovering."[43] In short, the process of gaining psychological knowledge through the 'sensus interiores' is suspected of being merely speculative. This is also the reason why self-observation, which was to play such a significant role in Karl Philipp Moritz's (1756–1793) *Psychologia empirica* (an experiential psychology characteristic of the late Enlightenment), is ignored by Krüger.[44] However, "physiognomy, which," according to

---

die Erfahrung mit der Vernunft, und diese mit jener verbinden."

[40] Krüger, *Experimental=Seelenlehre,* § 3, 4f: "Sind also nicht diejenigen, welche mit gänzlicher Hindansetzung aller sinnlichen Begriffe bloß der Vernunft folgen wollen, denen Kindern ähnlich, welche zu fahren hoffen, wenn sie in einem unbespannten Wagen die Sprache des Fuhrmanns nachmachen." "Ohne dieselbe [= Erfahrung; C.Z.] ein Naturlehrer werden zu wollen, heißt zur Befriedigung seiner Neubegierde eine Reise mit verbundenen Augen unternehmen."

[41] *Ibid.*, § 5, 13.

[42] Manfred Frank, *Selbstgefühl* (Frankfurt am Main 2002).

[43] Krüger, *Experimental=Seelenlehre,* § 5, 13 f.

[44] Cf. Karl Philipp Moritz, "Aussichten zu einer Experimentalseelenlehre" [1782], in Karl Philipp Moritz, *Werke,* ed. Horst Günther, vol. 3: *Erfahrung, Sprache, Denken,* 2. ed. (Frankfurt am Main 1993), 85-99, esp. 92 f.

Krüger, "had been excluded from psychology far too soon," is an important factor in the methodological classification of observations.[45]

The ideal solution within the concept of empirical psychology is based on the 'external senses'. In this context, two *modi operandi* can be distinguished: observation and experiment, or *"observationes et experimenta."* Whereas observation "requires unimpaired senses, attention and, if applicable, an instrument to sharpen the senses" alone, as "the thing itself or the object, that should be observed, remains unaltered," the same does not hold true for experiments. Experiments transfer things to a condition, "that they would not have come into otherwise, hence we are forcing nature to show us what it actually intended to hide from us."[46] Krüger counts microscopes and spring scales among the instruments that sharpen one's observation skills; one means of transferring things to a different condition would be a vacuum pump. "Is it possible, however, to apply the vacuum pump to the psyche, to view its shape through magnifying glasses and to weigh its forces?" Krüger asks ostentatiously at the beginning of his introduction to the *Experimental Psychology*, which sought to teach its readers that observation and experiment are two different things.[47] Joseph Wright of Derby's (1734–1797) *An Experiment on a Bird in the Air-Pump* (1769) can be seen as emblematic for the concept of experiment in the eighteenth century. The vacuum pump experiment is also incorporated in the center of the frontispiece to the *Encyclopédie*.

At the same time, Andreas Elias Büchner (1701–1769) distinguished between experiment and observation in a similar manner. In his work, *Der vernünftig rathende und glücklich curirende Medicus* ("The Reasonably Advicing and Successfully Curing Doctor") in 2 volumes (1762/65), he dedicates an extensive chapter to the rules "one should observe when conducting medical experiments."[48] As Büchner claims: "If we wish to learn something about a thing we should either leave it in the condition

---

45) Krüger, *Experimental=Seelenlehre*, § 5, 14.
46) *Ibid.*, § 6, 15: "darein sie sonst nicht gekommen sein würden, und dadurch wir die Natur zwingen, uns das zu zeigen, was sie sich vorgesetzt hatte für unsern Augen zu verbergen."
47) *Ibid.*, § 1, 1: "Wird man aber wohl die Geister unter die Luftpumpe bringen, ihre Gestalten durch Vergrößerungsgläser erblicken, und ihre Kräfte abwägen können?"
48) Büchner, *Medicus*, II, 136-256.

it is already in or bring it into a state in which it has not been before."[49] The first aspect refers to an "experience of the immediate intellect." But while Krüger calls this experience "observation" (*observatio*), Büchner does not have an appropriate term for it. The second aspect is referred to as "experiment": "An experiment is hence nothing else than an experience one gains by transferring a thing to a different state in which it would not have come into otherwise." Büchner offers the following examples to explain this distinction. If one wishes to find out whether one's heart is beating, one only needs to put a hand on the chest, "because then one will feel its movements." As for experiments, if, on the other hand, one would like to see the movements of the heart—e.g., of a dog—with one's own eyes, "one needs to open its chest, hence transferring it to a condition it has not been in before." Likewise, the case of a physician who administers a "medicine to a patient in order to see whether it helps," is regarded by Büchner as a "medical experiment."[50]

Similarly, while Krüger developed a casuistic of the psychological experiment, Büchner considered "two aspects" of medical experiments; namely, their "medical and their moral use." In this context, Büchner discusses experiments that are "morally evil," but "still beneficial from a medical point of view." He alludes here to Albrecht von Haller's methodical serial experiments conducted in Göttingen. Büchner specifies the case of a man, "for example, who sacrifices an entire flock of animals to prove something that he has invented in endless experiments."[51] Krüger also considers psychological human experiments but lets the "voice of humanity" object.[52] Though discussing experiments on delinquents and animals, he substitutes these for case reports, meaning by this the obser-

---

49) *Ibid.*, 228: "Wenn wir demnach in einer Sache etwas erfahren wollen, so lassen wir sie entweder in dem Zustande, darinnen sie sich befindet, oder wir versetzen sie in einen Zustand, darinnen sie vorher nicht war."

50) *Ibid.*, 228: "Ein Versuch ist also nichts anders, als eine Erfahrung, welche man erlangt, indem man ein gewisses Ding in einen Zustand setzet, in welchen es von sich selbst nicht gekommen wäre. [...] da er sodann das Schlagen des Herzens empfinden wird. [...] so muß er die Brust des Hundes eröfnen, und folglich denselben in einen Zustand versetzen, darinnen er vorher nicht war. [...] ein Arzneimittel eingiebt, um zu sehen, ob dieses demselben werde Hilfe verschaffen."

51) *Ibid.*, 231-32: "Wenn z.E. ein Mensch eine ganze Heerde von Thieren aufopfert, um dieses oder jenes, was er erfunden, durch unzählige Versuche zu bestätigen."

52) Krüger, *Experimental=Seelenlehre*, § 7, 18.

vation of the following instance in written form: If "incidentally"—e.g., due to an accident—"the psyche has been transferred to an exceptional and unusual state one can easily regard this as an experiment on the soul."[53] Krüger's work comprises of an extensive appendix that includes various case reports. Krüger hence substitutes experiments for a *casus* collection.[54] Here, we may indeed recognize the path that was to lead to Moritz's *Journal of Experiential Psychology* being paved.

3. 'Reforging' Man—the Anthropoietics of the 'Reasonable Physicians'

As we have seen, Hoffmann's concept of *observatio* is systematically ambiguous; it is at the same time an event and narration and an observation and discursive documentation—a fact that yields a peculiar reversal. It is not that the observation is documented in written form but that the rules of its documentation determine what it is that should actually be observed. The 'factum', as Joseph Vogl insists, is not what is given but rather what is created.[55] In regards to observation this holds true on three different levels.

A) By selecting significant events that are worth recording, a 'history of disease' is created. Like any other historiographer, the narrator of diseases is confronted with the challenge to choose only those aspects from the 'host' of events that are important for the course of disease. An "attentive physician" needs to observe "several minor things" that "might seem irrelevant to others." Büchner here systematically enhances Hoffmann's topic of a 'thorough' *historia morbi*, transforming it into a poetics of the case narrative in his chapter "About the Orderly Construction and Documentation of a Complete History of Disease, and

---

53) *Ibid.*, § 7, 20: "die Seele durch eine ausserordentliche Veränderung des Leibes in einen ausserordentlichen und ungewöhnlichen Zustand gerathen ist, daß man solche billig als Experimente, die mit der Seele angestellt worden sind, betrachten kann."
54) Cf. Zelle, „Experimentalseelenlehre und Erfahrungsseelenkunde"; Nicolas Pethes, *Zöglinge der Natur. Der literarische Menschenversuch des 18. Jahrhunderts* (Göttingen, 2007), 143-51, Tanja van Hoorn, "Stellers Seebär. Ein Anhang zur *Experimental-Seelenlehre* (1756)," in Alexander Košenina and Carsten Zelle, eds., *Kleine anthropologische Prosaformen der Goethezeit (1750–1830)* (Hannover, 2011), 51-66.
55) See Vogl, "Für eine Poetologie des Wissens," 114-15.

all the Parts that are Relevant for this."[56] At the same time, the 'attentive physician' must avoid "prolixity," for it is not necessary "to include all details and create a regular diary."[57] A mere string of events, however, does not make a *historia morbi*. One must know how to discern 'details' that are significant for the course of disease and those that are insignificant. Only those things "that are reasonably important" should be reported.[58] The narration should include only those aspects that are related to the respective disease which is characterized by a certain progression. According to Büchner every disease has its own "shape" and "order"; i.e., it corresponds to a specific "*typum*."[59]

Type of disease is the criterion that makes a single circumstance visible and communicable as a symptom, if applicable. Only within the interpretative frame of the "*typum*" does a circumstance become a symptom (or not, as the case may be). The observing physician sees himself confronted with a hermeneutic circle: To interpret a specific event as a symptom he must know the disease type; the disease type, however, is the result of the narrative string of individual events that show themselves as symptoms and are hence discernible from random incidents.

B) The topic of the *historia morbi* guides and channels the attention of the observing physician. The 'requisita' that Hoffmann defines as significant for a 'thorough' *observatio* should over time be cultivated into a dense topical network. These medical topoi not only classify the rhetorical disposition of the history of disease, but they also serve as a means to guide the physician's attention in the physical examination of the patient.

The patient's body, bodily functions as well as his or her mental and social condition are surveyed on the basis of a catalogue of questions that guide and condition the physician's attention. This guidance of attention refers to the exact empirical physical inventory and the precise documentation of the examination results stand in a close, reciprocal constitutional relationship with each other.

---

[56] Büchner, *Medicus*, I, 33–92 ("Von der ordentlichen Einrichtung und Aufzeichnung einer vollständigen Krankheits=Geschichte, und denen sämtlichen dazu erforderlichen Stücken"), § 5, 44.

[57] Büchner, *Medicus*, I, 33–92, § 18, 83.

[58] *Ibid.*

[59] *Ibid.*

C) The practice that patients submit their own case narratives to a doctor in the form of a letter to request a *consilium*, makes the self-exploring patient-writers become attentive explorers of their own self. Furthermore, this practice, which shall be dealt with below, sharpens and refines the 'sensus interior'. Ironically, self-observation, which had been described as unsuitable as a means of empirical data collection in Krüger's *Experimental Psychology* because of its affinity to the 'inner sense', is now unexpectedly revived in the frame of the epistolary consultation of doctors by their patients. So as to confirm the observation that this epistolary form of consultancy and its elevation to methodological statuete gave rise to the systematic self-observation of patients, I will turn briefly to Krüger's erstwhile student, the physician Johann August Unzer.

Unzer completed his studies in Halle and moved to the Danish town Altona to establish a flourishing practice. In his magazine, *Der Arzt*, he writes that many were involved in "corresponding" with him on their specific diseases to tell him their worries and to ask for his advice in writing.[60] Since the submitted accounts were mostly "too abstruse, obscure and insufficient" to give evidence about one's disease, Unzer developed a specific topic, almost a form of medical "confessional formula" or "form," pursuant to which patients should compile their medical reports. This "medical inquisition," as Unzer calls it ironically, includes a list of initially 16 and later 20 questions.[61] Unzer commits patients "to make themselves acquainted with the rules of how such a medical report should be prepared to ensure that the physician will be able to utter his advice and opinion in a proper manner."[62] In this context, Unzer emphatically defends the value of such medical reports against the "charlantanism" of uroscopy and other methods of formal medical semiotics.[63] In the frame of this consultation practice, patients are hence required to observe themselves pursuant to Unzer's topic. "Upon the origin and pro-

---

[60] Johann August Unzer, *Der Arzt. Eine medicinische Wochenschrift*, 12 vols. (Hamburg 1759–1764), vol. 7, 160st piece, 61-64, esp. 62.

[61] *Ibid.*, vol. 1, 9th piece, 129–44, esp. 135-37; vol. 7, 160st piece, 62-64. The later piece elaborates the further formular.

[62] *Ibid.*, vol. 7, 160st piece, 62: "ehe er eines entfernten Arztes Rath einholet, [sich] um die Regeln zu bekümmern, wie ein Krankenbericht an einen Arzt ordentlich einzurichten sey, damit er in Stand gesetzt werde, seinen Rath und seine Bedenken gründlich abzufassen."

[63] *Ibid.*, vol 1, 9th piece, 132.

gression of his disease," Unzer writes, "he will seek to optimize the explanations that he delivers to the doctor and that are based on the attentive observation of his nature, his lifestyle and his emotions."[64]

It is neither the churchly confession, nor the Pietist resurrection report, nor the sentimental diary that bring to light the subjective depths of the pre-romantic self. Instead, it is dietary questions such as: "11. Which emotions dominate a person? And how can the person cope with them?"[65] that create the self-referential loops of the modern sense of self.

The medical epistemology, which was developed by Hoffmann, Krüger, Büchner and other 'reasonable physicians' on the empirico-rationalistic basis of Wolff's philosophy, combined reason and experience, i.e. observation and experiment, with the technique of written narratives (*historia morbi*). Within the practice of letter-written *consilium*, as Unzer's case shows, this modell underwent a kind of subjective turn, because the observer was not longer the physician, but the patient itself. This process triggered *self*-observation and forced (in contrast to the former sceptical estimation, e.g. of Krüger) the nobilitation of *sensus interior*, which became the centre of a self-referential concept of the soul in the second part of the eighteenth century.[66]

---

[64] *Ibid.*, vol 1, 9th piece, 139: "durch eigene aufmerksame Beobachtung seiner Natur, seiner Lebensordnung und seiner Empfindungen beym ersten Ursprunge und beym Fortgange der Krankheit immer geschickte zu machen suchen, dem Arzte die Erläuterungen, die er bedarf, mitzutheilen."

[65] *Ibid.*, vol. 7, 160st piece, 63: "11. Welche Gemütsbewegungen beherrschen ihn? und wie faßt er sich darinn?".

[66] "Unsere Seele aber ist dasjenige Wesen, welches sich seiner selbst bewußt ist [...]." Albrecht von Haller, *Abhandlung von den empfindlichen und reizbaren Theilen des menschlichen Leibes* [lat. 1753], trans. Carl Christian Krause. Leipzig 1756, 22. Simon A.A.D. Tissot translates: "L'ame est cet être, qui se sent [...]." Albrecht von Haller, *Mémoires sur la nature sensible et irritable des parties du corps animal. Tome premier, contenant une seconde édition corrigée de la Dissertation sur l'irritabilité* [...], trans. Simon Auguste André David Tissot (Lausanne, 1756), 51. Cf. Rudolf Behrens, "'Sens intérieur' und meditierende Theoriesuche. Jacob Heinrich Meisters *Lettres sur l'imagination* (1794/1799)," in Peter-André Alt et al., eds., *Prägnanter Moment. Studien zur deutschen Literatur der Aufklärung und Klassik. Festschrift für Hans-Jürgen Schings* (Würzburg, 2002), 149-165. An extensive study of *sensus interior* in the mid 18th century lacks.—A modified german version of this paper appears as "Fall und Fallerzählungen in Friedrich Hoffmanns *Medicina Consultatoria* (1721-1739)," in Yvonne Wübben and Carsten Zelle, *Krankheit schreiben. Aufzeichnungsverfahren in Medizin und Literatur* (Göttingen, 2013), 348-73.

Writing Cases and Casuistic Reasoning in Karl Philipp Moritz' *Journal of Empirical Psychology*

Yvonne Wübben

*Ruhr-Universität Bochum**

Abstract

This paper examines medical writing in Karl Philipp Moritz' *Journal of Empirical Psychology* by looking at the alterations Moritz made to his sources. It shows how he rearranged the data in order to introduce a new type of text into psychology: the case or case study. He did so by altering the main parts of a report that had been published a few years earlier. In rewriting the report, Moritz introduced not only a new type of text but also a style of reasoning; i.e. the casuistic form of thinking that became more widely acknowledged only later in the course of experiential psychology (*Erfahrungsseelenkunde*). The paper thus links writing techniques in psychology to the rise of a type of text and a new style of reasoning.

Keywords

writing cases, case studies, history of psychology, epistemic genre, observation, report, experiential psychology, styles of reasoning, casuistic approach

Karl Philipp Moritz' *Magazin zur Erfahrungsseelenkunde* (Journal of Empirical Psychology) is one of the best known and arguably most important psychological journals of the Enlightenment.[1] First published in

---

* Ruhr-Universität Bochum, Mercator Forschergruppe "Räume anthropologischen Wissens", Universitätsstr. 150, 44801 Bochum, Germany (yvonne.wuebben@rub.de). This paper is a translated and extended English version of Yvonne Wübben, "Vom Gutachten zum Fall. Die Ordnung des Wissens in Karl Philipp Moritz 'Magazin zur Erfahrungssee-lenkunde',," in Sheila Dickson, Stefan Goldmann, Christoph Wingertszahn, eds., *"Fakta, und kein moralisches Geschwätz." Zu den Fallgeschichten im "Magazin zur Erfahrungs-seelenkunde" (1783–1793)* (Göttingen, 2011), 140–58.

[1] *GNOTHI SAUTON oder Magazin zur Erfahrungsseelenkunde als ein Lesebuch für Gelehrte und Ungelehrte*, ed., Karl Philipp Moritz, 10 vols (Berlin, 1783–1793; reprint

1783, it brings together various articles dealing with particular incidents under headings such as *Seelenkrankheitskunde* (the 'study of diseases of the soul', or psychopathology) and *Seelenzeichenkunde* (the 'study of the signs of the soul', or psychosemiotics). The range of subjects covered is extremely broad and includes popular issues such as the question of ghosts. However, unlike the *Berlinische Monatsschrift* (Berlin monthly periodical), the Enlightenment project of Johann Erich Biester and Friedrich Gedike which likewise first appeared in 1783, this journal is not a vehicle for a critique of superstition or religion.[2] Its aim is rather to make a valuable contribution to experiential psychology. In addition to its thematic diversity, the journal brings together very different types of text. In his proposal, *Vorschlag zu einem Magazin einer Erfahrungs-Seelenkunde*, which was published in 1782 in *Deutsches Museum*, Moritz in fact explicitly named the kinds of text he was looking for. He called for 'reports', 'observations', 'experimental descriptions', 'news from former pedagogues', 'biographies', 'diaries', 'stories of recovery', the 'story of lunatics and fanatics', 'plays' (Shakespeare), 'good novels' and 'observations from the real world'.[3] The list includes medical as well as literary genres and is, however, very revealing with regard to the history of knowledge.[4] Genre categories, as historian Gianna Pomata has noted, are by no means mere notes in the margins of the history of knowledge. Rather, they reflect modes of thought and reasoning and thus have an important cognitive dimension. They can be understood as systems of knowledge which provide an underlying structure, allowing material to be sorted and integrated into a given framework.[5] Moreover, it is possible to derive from

---

1978/79); for key studies on the journal's significance. see: Raimund Bezold, *Popularphilosophie und Erfahrungsseelenkunde im Werk von Karl Philipp Moritz* (Würzburg, 1984); Lothar Müller, *Die kranke Seele und das Licht der Erkenntnis. Karl Philipp Moritz' Anton Reiser* (Frankfurt a. M., 1987); and Sybille Kershner, *Karl Philipp Moritz und die "Erfahrungsseelenkunde." Literatur und Psychologie im 18. Jahrhundert* (Herne, 1991).

[2] Yvonne Wübben, *Gespenster und Gelehrte. Zur ästhetischen Lehrprosa Georg Friedrich Meiers (1718–1777)* (Tübingen, 2007), 171-72.

[3] Karl Philipp Moritz, "Vorschlag zu einem Magazin einer Erfahrungs-Seelenkunde," in Karl Philipp Moritz, *Werke*, Heide Hollmer and Albert Meier, eds., vol. 1 (Frankfurt a. M., 1999), 796-98.

[4] Gianna Pomata, "Sharing Cases: The Observationes in Early Modern Medicine," *Early Science and Medicine*, 15 (2010), 193-236, at 194.

[5] Pomata, "Sharing Cases," 197.

them the conventions of thought and the intellectual *habitus* of entire groups. The genre *contradicentia*, for instance, refers to a culture of academic controversy. Titles such as *experimenta* or *practica*, on the other hand, suggest the increasingly practical orientation of the early modern age. Moreover, the cyclical spread of certain genres can indicate significant shifts in the prevailing knowledge system, as the example of the *observatio* shows.[6] As the name suggests, the *observatio* asserts independent observation as a relevant source of knowledge. This gives us an intimation of the new role it was to assume.[7]

Moritz too refers to observation as the central means of acquiring knowledge and as a genre. He also expresses himself in a type of text which is not explicitly mentioned in the introduction but which clearly gains importance during the rise of modern psychology, psychiatry and psychoanalysis: the case or case study.[8] This type of text can be linked to these disciplines, and, thus, to a certain style of reasoning. In Moritz' journal it also corresponds to specific writing techniques, as this article seeks to demonstrate

Moritz not only obtained, collected and categorised the genres outlined above. He also revised existing genres—such as reports—to a considerable extent by altering main parts of the text, something which has not yet been investigated in depth. In the following, I will show how Moritz creates a 'case' (*Kasus*) from a medical report, thus reorganising the data in terms of the text-type 'case'.[9] When speaking here of 'case', the term is used partly in the sense proposed by André Jolle, according to whom a case represents a norm conflict and is determined by the opposition of the general and the particular. I will use the term in the same sense, but—in contrast to Jolles—as a descriptive category and not to

---

[6] Michael Stolberg, "Formen und Funktionen medizinischer Fallberichte in der Frühen Neuzeit," in Johannes Süßmann, Susanne Scholz and Gisela Engel, eds., *Fallstudien: Theorie—Geschichte—Methode* (Berlin, 2007), 81–95.

[7] Gianna Pomata, "Observation Rising. Birth of an Epistemic Genre, ca. 1500–1650," in Lorraine Daston and Elizabeth Lunbeck, eds., *Histories of Scientific Observation* (Chicago, 2011), 45-80.

[8] John Forrester, "If p, then What? Thinking in Cases," *History of the Human Sciences*, 9 (1996), 1–25.

[9] André Jolles, "Kasus," in André Jolles, *Einfache Formen. Legende, Sage, Mythen, Rätsel, Spruch, Kasus, Memorabile, Märchen, Witz* (Halle, 1956)Jolles, "Kasus," 141–164.

denote a 'simple form'.[10] While it is, of course, anachronistic to draw on Jolles' typology—Moritz does not use the term *Kasus* at all—it nevertheless allows us to view Moritz' alterations to the texts as deliberate revisions which create a new type of text and pursue a representational objective. This 'work on the genre'—i.e. reworking the medical report as a 'case'—expresses a desire to generalise and, it will be argued, a 'casuistic norm conflict' is enacted. Unlike in the medical report, the focus is no longer on an individual case but on the rule which this case represents. The genre's knowledge claim is not derived solely from the content, but also from the manner of representation. The latter reflects the development of certain modes of thought or styles of reasoning which were becoming central to empirical psychology.

The Story of the Spanish Weaver: from Medical Report to Case

Moritz' revision strategies are clearly recognisable in an item from 1783 about the 'disease of the mind' of a Spanish weaver. The article is based on the medical report of the Berlin city physician Johann Theodor Pyl (1749–1794). It discusses the case of a weaver who believed that spirits and angels had shown him the location of a treasure in the cellar of an acquaintance. When he got to the cellar, however, he was unable to find the treasure and became firmly convinced that it had been deliberately kept from him. He believed that his acquaintance had misappropriated it with criminal intent. It can no longer be ascertained in detail why the case was investigated officially and what prompted the call for a medical report examining the weaver's mental state. According to §220 of the Prussian Civil Code, *phantasmoscopia*—like other practices deemed su-

---

[10] On the medical case history in the early modern era (albeit without any definition of the genre), see Johanna Geyer-Kordesch, "Medizinische Fallbeschreibungen und ihre Bedeutung in der Wissensreform des 17. und 18. Jahrhunderts," *Medizin, Gesellschaft und Geschichte*, 9 (1990), 7–19, who relates its popularity to the forms of observation arising with cosmology and the study of natural history; a different view is presented by Müller, *Die kranke Seele*, 1–7, who emphasises the memorative function. On the poetics of the case history, see Carsten Zelle, "'Die Geschichte bestehet in einer Erzählung'. Poetik der medizinischen Fallerzählung bei Andreas Elias Büchner (1701–1769)," *Zeitschrift für Germanistik*, 19/2, (2009), 301–316.

perstitious—was punishable by imprisonment provided that mental confusion could be excluded.[11] The report may have formed part of criminal proceedings in which the man's mental state was examined. Of interest here is not so much the incident itself as the two surviving texts, Pyl's report and the article published in the *Journal*. I will begin by outlining these in greater detail.

Moritz relates the facts of the case in a four-page article entitled "The story of the disposition of Christian Philipp Schönfeld, a Spanish weaver in Berlin." The text consists of four sections. It begins with an introduction in which the editor refers to his source, namely Pyl's medical report. This is followed by a section providing general information about the mental disorder in question. The third section describes the sequence of events from the perspective of the person involved, and is followed, in a fourth section, by a conclusion. This structure itself is revealing—it is significant that the particulars of the case are preceded by a general psychological reflection on pathological states. Before coming to the actual facts, Moritz formulates a general rule:

> Constantly sitting in a hunched position, frequent and intense contemplation, and extensive recalculation in the case of difficult and artificial patterns, causes almost all people working at the loom to suffer from hypochondria and other concomitant complaints. If they also have a very lively temperament, it is all the more likely that a tendency to devise all manner of ventures and schemes ('project-making') may develop. The mind often suffers as a result, and, over time, particularly if the individual experiences hardship or misfortune, idiocy or actual insanity may ensue.[12]

According to this rule, virtually all weavers suffer from hypochondria, because they spend a lot of time seated at the loom. This hypochondria

---

[11] I would like to thank Bettina Wahrig (Technische Universität Braunschweig, Abteilung für Pharmazie- und Wissenschaftsgeschichte) for pointing this out to me.

[12] Moritz, "Gemüthsgeschichte Christian Philipp Schönfelds, eines spanischen Webers in Berlin," *Magazin zur Erfahrungsseelenkunde*, 1 (1783), 21: "Das beständige krumme Sitzen, oft scharfes Nachdenken, und weitläuftiges Ueberrechnen bei schweren und künstlichen Mustern, veranlaßt fast alle die Leute, welche auf dem sogenannten Stuhl arbeiten, zur Hypochondrie und daraus entspringenden Uebeln. Ist nun vollends ihr Temperament sehr lebhaft, so entsteht um so leichter ein Hang zum Projektmachen, wobei nicht selten der Verstand leidet, und mit der Zeit, besonders wenn sie noch in Noth und Unglück gerathen, Blödsinn, oder würklicher Wahnsinn entstehet."

becomes pathological under certain circumstances which may stem from the character of the individual (temperament) and/or events (hardship, misfortune). Moritz now follows this rule with more details about the weaver's life and character:

> The notion of hunting for treasure probably first came to our Schönfeld as a result of a propensity for idleness and a reluctance to work. Constantly thinking about this idea made such a strong impression on his already extremely lively imagination that it became a constant preoccupation. He created a dream for himself, which he gradually began to mistake for reality. This was already enough to confuse his mind. Illness, extreme hardship and distress followed. These completely unhinged his mind, and his sense of truth was now so dulled that he became firmly convinced of the reality of the following delusions.[13]

Moritz both stresses the weaver's propensity for idleness and outlines the course of his thoughts. These remarks are intended to further elucidate the rule or general principle. They describe how normal hypochondria can become pathological under certain circumstances. We can see from the additional remarks that individual elements, generally formulated in abstract terms only, take concrete form in the story of the weaver's life and are considered in relation to one another. When he mentions the weaver's "idleness" and his "reluctance to work," Moritz gives reasons for the pathological development which stem from the character of the individual. Idleness and sloth are, in the broadest sense, among the characteristics which were recognised as risk factors for the development of hypochondria. Hunting for treasures, on the other hand, is considered "project-making." According to Moritz, this is encouraged by a lively temperament and an excitable imagination. It can turn into hypochondria, as is the case here, if the "dream becomes reality." The weaver believed

---

13) Moritz, "Gemüthsgeschichte," 21: "Unsern Schönfeld brachte wahrscheinlich eine Neigung zum Müssiggange und Unlust zu arbeiten, zuerst auf die Gedanken, Schätze zu graben. Beständiges Nachdenken darüber, drückte diese Idee seiner ohnedem schon äußerst lebhaften Einbildungskraft so fest ein, daß sie ihm am Ende beständig gegenwärtig war, und er sich selber einen Traum schuf, den er nach und nach anfing für Wirklichkeit zu halten. Dieß verwirrte schon seinen Verstand. Nun kam noch Krankheit, äußerste Nothdürftigkeit und Kummer hinzu; diese zerrütteten vollends denselben, und sein Wahrheitsgefühl war nun so abgestumpft, daß er sich von der Wirklichkeit folgender Einbildungen fest überzeugen konnte."

that real spirits had shown him a real treasure. In the present case, the delusion is exacerbated by the circumstances of poverty and distress and ultimately results in a mental disorder: the firm conviction that the spirits and treasure are real.

The passage presents an individual case to illustrate Moritz's above-cited rule. To use Jolles' terminology, it relates the general to the particular, the fate of the Spanish weaver. But the passage not only serves to illustrate the rule. It has a second function also: it appears to transgress the rule, or to broaden its scope. The text ends with an unexpected and almost comical twist when another person becomes involved. The weaver's sister was also asked to attend the consultation which Pyl conducted and on which he based his report. Instead of refuting her brother's statements, as may have been expected from the case history, she unexpectedly agreed with him. She, too, believed that the treasure and the spirits were real. Thus the sister, summoned as a witness to confirm her brother's insanity, in fact does the exact opposite.[14] Moritz concludes from this that insanity is contagious and thus generates a second rule which is not contained in the report. Pyl, the doctor, had spoken only of the sister's madness, not of contagion by madness.[15]

One is first struck by Moritz's numerous revisions to the original regarding the arrangement and framing of the material. He makes no secret of these; before presenting the case he introduces himself as the editor and states that he has "arranged the information, however, in terms of my intended purpose."[16] This remark may suggest that the readers of the *Journal* had a knowledge of textual history. Readers may indeed have been able to differentiate between a medical report and other types of text, such that it was only reasonable to inform them of any alterations. A comparison with Pyl's report shows that Moritz deviates from the genre of the medical report in two crucial points. He makes two changes to the sequence which alter the structure of the text and have a significant impact on its genre classification.

Pyl's text has a clear structure which largely conforms to the genre 'medical report'. It consists of a 'relatio' (i.e., the presentation of the case

---

[14] Johann Theodor Pyl, *Auffsätze und Beobachtungen aus der gerichtlichen Arzeneywissenschaft* (Berlin, 1784), 172–73.

[15] *Ibid.*, 173.

[16] Moritz, "Gemüthsgeschichte," 21.

and/or examination of the patient) and a 'ratio' (the actual medical opinion). These two main sections are also separated typographically in Pyl's
report.[17] Each main section is subdivided into further sections, which are
also separated typographically. The 'relatio' consists of five sections. The
first section begins by stating the time, the place and the persons involved in the examination. This is followed by a paragraph describing the
content of the examination and the observations made. It begins as follows:

> He was initially fairly relaxed. As soon as we came to the topic of the treasure hunt
> and the two hundred million that were found, he became heated. We presented to
> him repeatedly and in different ways the improbability of his claim; that it was
> impossible that such a large sum had been found and that this could remain con-
> cealed, as he himself maintained that so many people had known of it. Further-
> more, his statement was made all the more improbable as he had not spoken out
> sooner. After all, as he himself admitted, this treasure had been found as early as
> 1764, and he allegedly knew that part of it had been transferred to Potsdam. How
> was it possible that he could determine so precisely the value of the same, when
> he himself admitted that he had not seen any of it, but only, according to his report,
> tightly closed crates, barrels and pots containing the treasure; he, however, had not
> seen what was contained therein, nor even lifted them himself?—whether it was
> not the case that his imagination and fantasy, which by his own admittance
> deceived him so often, had not misled him here also?[18]

---

[17] On reconstructing the facts in (legal) reports, see Konstantin Imm, "Zur Einführung
in den Gegenstandsbereich," in Jörg Schönert, ed., *Erzählte Kriminalität. Zur Typologie
und Funktion von narrativen Darstellungen in Strafrechtspflege, Publizistik und Literatur
zwischen 1770 und 1920* (Tübingen, 1991), 21.

[18] Pyl, *Auffsätze*, 168–73: "Anfangs war er ziemlich gelassen, sobald wir aber auf den
Punkt des Schatzgrabens und der gefundenen zweyhundert Millionen kamen, ward er
hitzig, und ob wir ihm gleich verschiedentlich und wiederholentlich das Unwahrschein-
liche seines Vorgebens vorstelleten, wie es unmöglich sey, daß eine so grosse Summe
gefunden sey und solches verschwiegen bleiben könne, da er doch behauptet, daß so
viele Leute Wissenschaft davon gehabt hätten; wie ferner seine Angabe dadurch um so
unwahrscheinlicher würde, daß er sich nicht ehre gemeldet, da doch, wie er selbst
gestand, dieser Schatz schon 1764 gefunden worden, und er angeblich gewußt, daß ein
Theil davon nach Potsdam geführt würde, wie es möglich daß er so genau den Wehrt
dersselben bestimmen köne, da er doch selbst eingeständе, daß er nichts davon gesehen,
sondern blos seiner Angabe nach stark vermachte Kasten, Tönchen und Kessel, worinn
der Schatz enthalten gewesen, er aber das was darinn enthalten gewesen, nicht gesehen,
auch sie nicht einmahl selbst gehoben hätte?—ob nicht vielmehr seine Einbildung und

In addition to the observation of the psychological state (heated, relaxed), this passage also indirectly charts the course of the examination, which sought to impress on the weaver the absurdity and inconsistency of his claims.[19] This is followed by another paragraph containing another observation, namely that the interviewee was prone to contradict himself. The (corroborating) opinion is then cited of a parson who was involved in the matter.[20] He is quoted as saying that a moral factor (laziness) and a lively imagination could be considered reasons for searching for treasure. This opinion receives medical confirmation in the fifth paragraph. Here the doctor diagnoses the weaver's lively "temperament" on the basis of the "wild look in his eyes" and his "heart palpitations" and "anxiety."[21] Finally, the sixth paragraph formulates the rule, which Moritz also cites, that idleness may, under certain circumstances, lead to insanity. Pyl comes to the conclusion ('ratio') that the weaver is insane and thus confirms an existing suspicion. The final paragraph no longer conforms rigidly to the genre pattern of the medical report. Here the doctor mentions the weaver's sister, whom he likewise diagnoses with 'insanity'.

In Moritz's version, numerous passages of the report are deleted; others are elaborated or rearranged. The first passages to be deleted are those which refer to the specific examination situation and therefore contain observations and sentences which are formulated from the perspective of the interviewer ("I am wholly of the opinion that," "He was initially fairly relaxed").[22] More significant than the deletions, however, are the changes to the order; i.e., the rearrangement of individual sections. Moritz gives priority to the general rule with which Pyl had ended his report. It is now placed at the beginning. This also changes its textual function. The rule no longer supports the medical opinion, the 'ratio'. It can now be seen as a kind of instruction to the reader on how to interpret the following text. Moritz thus begins with the general statement under

---

Phantasie, die ihn wie wir ihn aus seinem eigenen Reden überführten, so oft täuschten, auch hier irre geführt hätten?"

[19] Pyl refers to evidence by inspection (*Auffsätze*, 69), which Stolberg makes the central criterion of the 'observationes'; cf. see Stolberg, "Formen und Funktionen," 81–95.

[20] Pyl's text contains a reference to a journal on which he was able to draw (*Auffsätze*, 169).

[21] Pyl, *Auffsätze*, 171–172.

[22] Pyl, *Auffsätze*, 168.

which the particular, the case of the weaver, is meant to be subsumed. This rearrangement can be understood as systematic 'work on the genre' inasmuch as it transforms the medical report into a case. It is only by virtue of this rearrangement—and this is the point at issue here—that Moritz's text can be categorised as a 'case'.[23] This is because the text now contains a component of the 'case', the general rule under which the particular is subsumed or for which it stands. A medical report arrives at an opinion in a specific case and explains this with the rule. By contrast, the 'case' begins by conveying the rule or general knowledge and then uses an individual instance to illustrate. The rearrangement thus indicates the creation of a case. Placing the rule at the beginning not only gives it a prominent position within the text, but also assigns it the function of making an event readable, subsuming it under something general and expressing generalisability. As a text-type, the 'case' thus has a grammar which is assigned to a paradigm. Unlike in a medical report, the specific facts are not of interest as an isolated instance, but rather because they can be subsumed and because they—like the example— function paradigmatically. It should be noted, however, that the paradigmatic function contains a contradiction which lies in the respective intrinsic validity of the general and the particular.[24] The general is an abstract rule which can never be wholly applied to the individual case. In turn, the individual case is invariably characterised by elements which are not covered by the rule. This results in a constitutive tension which can be detected to some extent in the choice of words. At the level of the word, transitions from the general to the particular take place, for instance, when Moritz gives the proper name ('Schönfeld')[25], which also provided the story's title.[26]

There is yet another indication that Moritz systematically modifies Pyl's report to create a case. The second significant alteration is at the end of the text. Here Moritz suggests that insanity is contagious and in so doing implicitly formulates a new rule. Moritz writes:

---

23) Jolles, "Kasus," 141–64.
24) Susanne Lüdemann, "Literarische Fallgeschichten. Schillers 'Verbrecher aus verlorener Ehre' und Kleists 'Michael Kohlhaas'," in Jens Ruchatz, Stefan Willer and Nicolas Pethes, eds., *Das Beispiel. Epistemologie des Exemplarischen* (Berlin, 2007), 208–23.
25) Moritz, "Gemüthsgeschichte," 11.
26) This is also true of Moritz's novel *Anton Reiser* (1785–90).

When the doctor and city physician Pihl [!] examined his state of mind on 18 June 1781, he was initially quite relaxed. However, as soon as we came to the topic of the treasure hunt and the two hundred million that were found, he became heated. Indeed, by his own admittance his imagination deceived him constantly, but there was no way of persuading him that the discovery of treasure itself was even remotely a delusion. Doctor Phil summoned his sister Cath. Elisab. Schönfeld in order to gain more insight from her regarding her brother's circumstances. She, however, confirmed all of her brother's foolish fantasies and was every bit as mad as he. Evidence of the experience that insanity is contagious.[27]

The story ends with a surprising twist, akin to a joke or *bon mot*.[28] It raises an unresolved aspect of the rule and thus contributes to a norm conflict, or to a further elaboration of the rule (e.g. in the sense that insanity can be contagious and that statements by third parties are only reliable if these have not themselves been infected with insanity). This second alteration likewise shapes the text in terms of the 'case'. As we know from Jolles, this consists not only in a rule, but also in the transgression of the rule. The case thus transmits an aspect which is not initially able to be subsumed under the rule.

In addition to this subsumption tendency, however, the text also tells an individual story. The language thus communicates the case of the weaver. Jolles himself addresses the "linguistic gesture" of the case when he concedes that every case only acquires substance through language, which always conveys more than the case itself.[29] The gesture embellishes the incident, creating calculated effects. Moritz devotes a lot of space to the weaver's words: they fill five separate paragraphs and occupy almost two thirds of the entire text. The text thus focuses on the

---

[27] Moritz, "Gemüthsgeschichte," 24: "Als der Herr Doktor und Stadtphysikus Pihl [!] den 18ten Junii 1781 seinen Gemüthszustand untersuchte, war er anfänglich ganz gelassen, sobald man aber auf den Punkt des Schatzgrabens und der gefundenen zweihundert Millionen kam, ward er hitzig. Man überführte ihn wirklich aus seinen eignen Reden, daß seine Phantasie ihn alle Augenblick täuschte, dahin aber war er auf keine Weise zu bringen, die Schatzhebung selber auch nur im mindesten für Täuschung zu halten. Der Herr Doktor Pihl ließ seine Schwester Cath. Elisab. Schönfeld zu sich kommen, um über die Umstände ihres Bruders mehr Licht von ihr zu erhalten. Diese aber bekräftigte alle thörichten Einbildungen ihres Bruders wörtlich, und war völlig so närrisch, wie er. Ein Beleg zu der Erfahrung, daß der Wahnwitz ansteckt."

[28] Of note are also the syntactic ambiguities arising from the use of the pronoun 'he'.

[29] Jolles, "Kasus," 141–64.

weaver's perspective. Moritz repeatedly regulates the distance to the protagonist through his choice of words when he describes the weaver as
"our Schönfeld."[30] This kind of effect may be achieved not only through
attributive embellishments, but also by the narrative. One of the frequently used, specifically narrative strategies is the successive reduction
of mediacy. This can be reconstructed in detail in the present example.
The text begins with a general observation which can be ascribed to the
editor. It underscores his authority, provides an overview and includes a
commendation of the city physician. The framing introduction is separated by a dash, signalling a change of speaker. Moritz no longer speaks
as editor and publisher of the text, but proceeds to the account of the
incident with a summary characterisation of Schönfeld. The incident is
then recounted straightforwardly in indirect speech (that of the weaver);
the account is much closer to the experience of the protagonist ("He
believed without a doubt that ...").[31] It acquires still greater immediacy
in the following through the omission, over extensive passages, of *verba
dicendi* ("The saints and spirits have revealed it to him").[32] Some of these
passages have been taken verbatim from Pyl. However, they no longer
fulfil the function of providing evidence as they had in the medical report. They describe details which are not essential to an understanding
of the rule.[33] These passages therefore point to a literary narrator who
seeks to entertain and whose shaping of the material is guided by aes-
thetic concerns.[34]

As we have seen, Moritz's case descriptions fall back on certain literary
techniques. For instance, a viewpoint must be chosen from which the
story is told, and this invariably casts the subject matter in a certain light.
Even the most 'objective' story depends on these techniques. This distin-

---

[30] Moritz, "Gemüthsgeschichte," 11.

[31] *Ibid.*, 22.

[32] *Ibid.*

[33] Robert Leventhal, "Vorstudien zur Hysterie. Marcus Herz' 'Etwas Psychologisches-
Medizinisches'. Moriz Krankengeschichte (1798)," in Ulrich Johannes Schneider, ed.,
Kulturen des Wissens im 18. Jahrhundert (Berlin, 2008), 431-440, 432.

[34] Nicolas Pethes, "Vom Einzelfall zur Menschheit. Die Fallgeschichte als Medium der
Wissenspopularisierung zwischen Recht, Medizin und Literaturm," in Gereon Blaseio,
Hedwig Pompe and Jens Ruchatz, eds., *Popularisierung und Popularität* (Cologne, 2005),
63-92, 70.

guishes the case from the medical report, which does not tell a story but rather, strictly speaking, recounts stories that have already been told.

To sum up, Moritz reworks the medical report as a case. He deviates from the original text by placing the rule at the beginning. Furthermore, Moritz adds a humorous twist and thus transgresses the rule. The revision takes place in the interest of a twofold tendency which both subsumes the case under a general statement and, in so doing, expresses a desire to generalise. It remains open, however, how this desire to generalise is justified and on which universal psychological laws the rule is actually based.

'Erfahrungsseelenkunde' and Enlightenment Psychology

Moritz' case is anchored in a pre-existing knowledge system which formulates just such universal psychological laws and which provides a broader interpretive framework (which, however, Moritz does not discuss). Similarities become apparent if we compare the above example of the Spanish weaver with thematically related Enlightenment texts. Many of the articles on the *Journal* draw on knowledge from empirical Enlightenment psychology. A passage from Georg Friedrich Meier's 1747 treatise on ghosts, *Gedancken von Gespenstern*, illustrates this:

> This person [the one who sees ghosts; YW] lies alone at night in his room. He hears measured steps, slow and heavy, outside his door. Here he has a clear sensation. Now, as he does not have a clear sensation of the cause of these steps and, moreover, has heard many tales of ghosts that creep around houses at night [...], he sees some similarity between his sensation and a ghost; as a consequence, he takes [...] his sensation to be the appearance of a ghost. His imagination now becomes heated. A thousand fearful images present themselves to his mind. His blood is thrown into confusion and he is seized by terrible emotions. If the imagination now becomes delirious, there is almost no way of stopping it. These illusions then acquire such a degree of clarity and force that they are taken for sensations, and a person can believe he has seen and heard things whose reality exists only inside his head.[35]

---

[35] Georg Friedrich Meier, *Gedancken von Gespenstern* (Halle, 1747), 8: "Dieser Mensch [der Gespensterseher; YW] liegt des Nachts allein in seiner Kammer. Er hört vor der Kammerthür abgemessene starcke und langsame Schritte. Hier hat er eine klare Empfindung. Da er nun die Ursache dieser Schritte nicht klar empfindet und da er nun

Here we have once more someone seeing phantoms. A man is in his room at night. He hears steps, not knowing where they are coming from, and believes he is seeing a ghost. His imagination is set in motion and the illusion becomes reality. Unlike Moritz, Meier relates specific individual observations with psychological concepts. The description of a mental process ("hearing steps") is followed by a general psychological concept ("clear sensation"). Description and general concepts are directly interwoven. Meier's text begins with a perception which is described in the terminology of Enlightenment psychology as 'clear sensation' ("He hears measured steps, slow and heavy, outside his door. Here he has a clear sensation"). An internal psychological process is conveyed by a concept. Furthermore, the example demonstrates that the imagination can produce illusions that are confused with perceptions and that this confusion is fostered not only by the imagination but also by a lively temperament.[36] An excessive imagination is mentioned as the chief factor in "seeing ghosts." In this passage, Meier thus gives an example for the pathology of the imagination that relies on his preconceived concepts of the lower senses and their function. At the same time, he remains vague as to how the 'heated' imagination contributes to the confusion. However, Meier's account does not discuss a medical case. It illustrates various mental processes using the Enlightenment approach, which claims to know how human consciousness functions and thus to be able to distinguish false-

---

überdies eine gantze Menge von Gespenstern aus der Erzählung anderer weiß, die des Nachts in den Häusern herumschleichen [...], so sieht er einige Aehnlichkeit zwischen seiner Empfindung und einem Gespenste; folglich hält er [...] seine Empfindung für die Erscheinung eines Gespenstes. Hierauf wird seine Einbildungskraft erhitzt. Tausend fürchterliche Bilder stellen sich seinem Gemüthe dar. Sein Geblüt kommt in Unordnung, und er wird von den entsetzlichsten Gemüthsbewegungen hin und her getrieben. Fängt die Einbildungskraft einmal an zu schwärmen: so kann man ihr kaum Einhalt thun. Diese Vorstellungen erlangen dadurch einen solchen Grad der Klarheit und der Stärcke, daß sie für Empfindungen gehalten werden, und daß ein Mensch glauben kann, er habe Dinge gesehen und gehört, die blos in seinem Kopfe ihre Würcklichkeit haben."

[36] Meier develops a total of three psychological/medical opinions on seeing ghosts. He attributes it to a structural imbalance between sensation and imagination, to a deception of the lower sensory faculties and, thirdly, to a nervous impulse. Meier accompanies these three options with a series of brief stories which have an illustrative function and can be understood as a narrative of *phantasmoscopia*; for more details see Wübben, *Gespenster*, 14.

hood from true sensation. Between Meier's treatise on ghosts and Moritz' journal lie more than forty years in which experiential psychology was less and less influenced by the methods of philosophical psychology. But there are still numerous parallels and common features that seem to be worth mentioning. First of all, both Moritz and Meier hold similar mechanisms responsible for false perceptions. Moritz likewise attributes the seeing of ghosts to a lively imagination.[37] His argument is based on concepts of 'imagination', 'insanity' and 'illusion', which are independent of experience. It is thus founded on knowledge that is valid irrespective of the concrete example, and grounded in Enlightenment philosophical psychology. But there are also obvious differences in the style of reasoning that can be linked to writing cases. Whereas Meier refers to a single incident—a person who sees ghosts—he does not mention a general rule or reflect on its applicability to the single instance. Taking this into account, Moritz' text can be connected to a style of reasoning that became crucial for psychology only later in its course; i.e., making a connection between a single particular instance and a general rule. Moritz connects both in a twofold way. The pre-existing rule is applied to the single incident as well as the single incident leads to a new rule.[38] Whereas Meier makes use of the ghost-seer only as an example for the mechanisms of the imagination, Moritz tries to derive knowledge from the particular. In this attempt, he follows a casuistic style of reasoning.

Despite of this new style of reasoning, almost all of the stories in the *Journal* about people who see ghosts draw—as I mentioned before—on a conceptual framework concerning the governing of mental processes. Philosophical Enlightenment psychology with its preconceived notions and knowledge of the universal is still present in his journal and remains influential in the field of knowledge as it determines the contents of the empirically-minded journal. One might almost say that it is with this prior knowledge that the events are able to be narrated at all or are made

---

[37] Meier, *Gedancken*, 14.

[38] There is no tendency to describe the individual in its very individuality. This is a main aspect of 'clinical writing' that Foucault and—following him—Andreas Gailus have pointed out; see Michel Foucault, *Discipline and Punish* (London, 1977), 191, and Andreas Gailus, "A Case of Individuality: Karl Philipp Moritz and the Magazine for Empirical Psychology," *New German Critique. An Interdisciplinary Journal of German Studies*, 79 (2000), 67–105.

plausible.[39] Universal philosophical definitions that were already in place around 1750 are to a large extent still inherent in the journal's narrations. From a theoretical perspective such a kind of universalism must be in conflict with the experiential, casuistic approach. Yet this seems no issue for the author. The concepts are juxtaposed with rules which are demonstrated or amplified on the basis of individual observations. Apparently, the approach is not underpinned by a terminology of its own. Its style of reasoning is mainly reflected by the text-type 'case', which is the result of a systematic textual revision.

---

[39] Georg Eckardt, "Anspruch und Wirklichkeit der Erfahrungsseelenkunde, dargestellt an Hand periodisch erscheinender Publikationen um 1800," in Olaf Breidbach and Paul Ziche, eds., *Naturwissenschaften um 1800. Wissenschaftskultur in Jena-Weimar* (Weimar, 2001), 179–202.

Index nominum

Index rerum

Printed in the United States
by Baker & Taylor Publisher Services